The Divine Connection

Dr. Donald Whitaker
with Bill Keith

HUNTINGTON HOUSE, INC.
1200 N. MARKET
SHREVEPORT, LOUISIANA 71107
(318) 222-1350

Bill Keith is a state senator from Louisiana and also is a free-lance writer. He lives in Mooringsport, Louisiana.

Introduction

I have known Dr. Whitaker since soon after he was miraculously healed on his deathbed and became a follower of Jesus Christ.

Having almost destroyed his own life, he was saved from a premature and needless early death. With a new lease on life through God's mercy, Dr. Whitaker snapped to attention and his penetrating and calculating mind began to re-analyze and to review this life from a new perspective.

Dr. Whitaker made the simple, yet profound discovery that human persons are created in God's image and that the faculties and functions of the human body are made for health, happiness and longevity — if the sensible basics of God's nature and his life-style are interwoven. These constitute what the Doctor calls the DIVINE CONNECTION.

But with Divine creation came human freedom. Dr. Whitaker learned that God gave to every person the sacred, inviolable right of *choice* to do good or bad, to abuse or to preserve oneself. People are free to self-destruct if they choose. Human persons can commit quick, or slow suicide. They can do it with a rope, a gun — or a life-style of wrong eating practices, abusive physical habits, destructive mental attitudes, inadequate exercise, lack of rest, hyper-recreational tendencies, etc.

Dr. Whitaker, a specialist in the science of the human anatomy, knows the miraculous regenerative and preservative powers that are inherent in every physical body. Medical Science has been telling us everywhere that we are made for health and longevity — at least for 120-140 productive years of good life.

Having been given a second chance at life, by God's miracle intervention in Dr. Whitaker's body when he was beyond the help of medical science, he discovered God, then God's wonderful health plan with its simple rules for a long and good life.

With a passion to help people enjoy this life and not destroy it, he re-launched his whole professional career toward teaching people the easy and sensible rules to happy, healthy and long living.

Dr. Whitaker saw the DIVINE CONNECTION.
  That gave him the lead to God's direction.
It provides you now with new projection
  To lift you out of your imperfection.

It offers you renewed circumspection
   With the right degree of introspection,
To help you make the right detection
   And give you God's guaranteed protection.

It removes the curse of deep abjection
   Or abusive, poisonous self-dejection;
It breaks the yoke of forced subjection,
   Prejudice, fear and self-rejection.

Doc saw that with some basic correction,
   Aided by God's renewed perfection,
You would make the right selection
   And discover the power of DIVINE CONNECTION.

— By T.L. Osborn

Dedication

Dedicated to my two sons —
Eric Eugene and Troy Lee.
They gave meaning to my life
and the desire to live
the many times that I did not wish to live
before I met Jesus.
They continue to bless my life now.

Contents

Contents

Preface

Dr. Donald Whitaker is a man with an unusual calling on his life — to help God's people have good health, enjoy life and live longer. Reading through the pages of this book you will discover a magnificent blueprint for that kind of life.

This doctor has received special insight and vision from the Lord concerning the cause-effect relationship between life-style and poor health. His basic premise is that we are a nation of sick people because of the way we eat and a diet that includes a lot of poison additives, preservatives, fat and sugar.

He says there are three basic reasons for this crisis in the lives of the American people. They include:

1. The way we eat.
2. The food we eat.
3. Our life-styles in general.

He says we are digging our graves with our teeth.

According to Dr. Whitaker, each year the average American consumes 120-130 pounds of white sugar; 88 pounds of white flour; 53 pounds of refined fats and oils; 14 pounds of processed corn; and seven pounds of white rice.

And, he says: "There is very little food value in any of these things for approximately 98 percent of the nutrients have been destroyed before they reach the dinner table."

Dr. Whitaker also points out that there are about 10,000 chemicals, emulsifiers and other different flavor enchanting additives in the foods that we eat. Some are known carcinogenics; yet we continue to eat them largely due to ignorance and indifference.

He believes the American people should be tired of feeling bad because of the kinds of food we eat and should be ready to make a change.

He says that people really want to change but don't know how.

According to Dr. Whitaker, we must get our priorities in order. We can continue to eat the wrong foods, refuse to exercise, fail to deal with stress and die young. Or, we can change our life-styles by eating properly, getting plenty of exercise and live long, fruitful lives — only after we get our systems back in order.

"But the choice is yours," he says. "No one can make that choice for you."

Dr. Whitaker, who was miraculously healed on a death bed, builds a strong biblical case for total health through self-discipline. He knows God's perfect plan is Divine health over Divine healing. God's Word says God's perfect plan is Divine health over Divine healing.

"Bless God He healed me — but I know God did

not want me sick in the first place," he says. "It was my fault."

God cannot make you sick for it goes against His Word, Dr. Whitaker says.

He points out that God's Word says: "Keep thy heart with all diligence; for out of it are the issues of life" (Proverbs 4:23).

There is a distinct spiritual dimension in good health, he says.

"A person cannot be at peace with himself if he does not have peace with God and one cannot have good health unless he has peace with himself," Dr. Whitaker says. "People who don't feel good may not feel close to God for there is a DIVINE CONNECTION between spirituality and good health."

People must be disciplined in order to have good health and to feel good, he says, and they must learn to push back from the table, say no to the wrong foods, and learn to exercise the body.

"Obedience is better than sacrifice and without discipline you cannot have obedience," he says. "Some people think that Satan can make you sick but Satan cannot make you sick unless you give him place."

The doctor says there are seven basic tenets to good health:

1. Correct eating habits.
2. Correct vitamins and minerals.
3. Adequate sleep and rest.
4. A regular program of exercise.
5. Adequate intake of pure water.
6. A positive outlook on life.
7. A changing of life-style.

By following these proven principles nearly anyone can develop:

1. More physical energy.
2. A sharper mind.
3. A better memory.
4. Calmness.
5. Coolheadedness.
6. Self-control.
7. Better looks.

Those who refuse the disciplined life-style, he
says, will experience the opposite, feeling:

1. Half dead.
2. Doped with stimulants and prescription
   medicines.
3. Irritable.
4. Tired and sluggish.
5. Little self esteem.

"Some people are in such poor health, they are
essentially already dead — they are just sleep-
walking," he says.

After a 17-year-practice of orthodox medicine as a
physician and surgeon, Dr. Whitaker turned his practice around to Orthomolecular and Preventive Medicine.

"By orthodox medicine I mean that I used the
three modalities such as medicine, surgery or radia-
tion which would include X-ray therapy for the treatment of disease," he says. "However, I discovered I
was going about medicine backwards. Orthodox
medicine waits until the patient becomes ill before

treating him. I now practice preventive medicine which means preventing disease rather than treating it. I can treat cancer, heart disease and other illnesses — or, I can prevent them in the majority of cases. I know God's best is Divine health.''

Dr. Whitaker also says that at creation God started the human body out the way He wanted it. Now he wants it back the way He started it.

After only six years in preventive medicine, Dr. Whitaker is beginning to receive calls from doctors throughout the land who have become interested in the wellness movement.

''Some of them have been watching my practice for several years and want to know what I'm doing and how I'm doing it,'' he says.

Dr. Whitaker notes that Thomas Edison, the great inventor, more than 50 years ago made a very astute observation on the role of the doctor of the future.

''The doctor of the future will give no medicine, but will interest his patients in the care of the human frame and diet and the cause and the prevention of disease,'' Edison said.

Dr. Whitaker has shared his insight with a large segment of the American people through his periodic appearances on the Trinity Broadcasting Network, The 700 Club, the PTL Club and other programs. He has a weekly television program that is seen coast to coast three times a week. And, his far-reaching health concepts have been well received by audiences everywhere.

He also holds Total Health Seminars and crusades all over America.

There have been thousands of books written on

disease, but very few on the prevention of disease. This is one of those books.

— *Bill Keith*

CHAPTER 1

Whatever Became of Good Health?

The Fountain of Youth syndrome exists in everyone causing them to want to feel better and live longer.

You can — through Divine health.

Americans in general, and Christians in particular, are overweight, out of shape and burned out physically and emotionally.

Whatever became of good health? We threw it away!

The truth is that the body of Christ is sick. Instead of feeling like a million, as God intended, most Christians feel like they are a million years old. Rather than living on the mountaintop of good health, most are just surviving in the valley of sickness.

I believe God's perfect will is for his people to be in good health and feel good all the time. That is the way he created us. He made our marvelous bodies to work and function perfectly.

Yet many Christians are overweight, tired, listless, irritable, depressed, weak and have a general case of the blahs. They have headaches, backaches, allergies, insomnia and a host of other problems. These ultimately lead to chronic illness, despondency and despair.

Some Christians grow old long before their time. They develop dry, wrinkled skin, fatigue, forgetfulness, and aches and pains.

Only the return of Christ or death can keep us from growing older. But Divine health can certainly keep us from looking and feeling older.

Did you know that God has a plan for total fitness and wellness? He has explained it to us in his Word.

God's plan and provision is for you to be well.

After training in some of the finest medical institutions in the world, I practiced orthodox medicine for 17 years. I was taught that if something couldn't be cured to just cut it out. My learned professors also told me that if I could not determine what was wrong with a patient that the patient must be suffering from psychosomatic or mental illness.

Yet instruction in the prevention of illness was sorely lacking in my medical training. It is still sorely lacking in most medical institutions in this United States.

The Prophet Hosea's ancient words of admonition are just as current as today's newspaper when he said: "My people are destroyed for lack of knowledge . . ." (Hosea 4:6).

God's people, for lack of knowledge, are destroying themselves today. They are digging their graves with their own teeth.

Many Christians have become just like the American government — big, fat and out of control.

One of my closest friends is a state senator in Oklahoma, a man who at one time was considered the second most powerful man in the state.

After I trusted Christ as savior, I shared my new faith with him hoping he would come over to our side.

The senator listened very intently to my testimony, then said, "I'm going to tell you how the world looks at Christians. They are usually overweight, always late for appointments and seldom pay their bills on time."

His analysis of Christians stunned, even shocked me. Then I started looking around and discovered there was a lot of truth in what he said.

During my 20 years as a physician and surgeon I have performed or assisted in surgery on hundreds of patients. It always amazed me when I took the scalpel and opened a patient's abdomen. What did I find? In a large number of patients we found that there was always an amazing amount of fat in the stomach area. There was also fat around blood vessels, around the intestines. I also noted while assisting on autopsies that a person who was overweight always had an increased amount of fat around the heart which accounted for many instances of congestive heart failure, enlargement of the heart, and heart disease in many forms.

Several years ago when God began leading me away from a practice of acute medicine and surgery into a practice of preventive medicine to help people stay well, I remembered that there is a saying in medicine that "health is wealth." We know that salvation from sin is the most important thing in life. However, after salvation next comes health for without health you cannot function as God ordained you to do.

Sir Francis Bacon, the eminent English philosopher and author, once said: "A healthy body is the guest chamber of the soul; a sick one, its prison."

The Lord began to show me that He has laws that relate to Divine health. Most people are born with good health but lose it when they break the natural laws of God.

The Spirit of God caused the Apostle John to write to the church: "Beloved, I wish above all things that thou mayest prosper and be in health, even as thy soul prospereth" (III John 2).

If our soul is not prospering and we are not in health we are going against His Word and are not in His Divine will.

God miraculously heals. He healed me of an incurable disease. While in Africa I saw dozens of blind people healed. I saw crippled people walk and cancer healed. Once I saw a little African boy with no eyeballs or sockets receive healing — first the sockets and then eyes. This was during a T.L. Osborn crusade in Kenya in 1978. I checked the child again in 1979 and the child had perfect vision.

Yes, God miraculously heals. His healing is as real today as it was in the time of Jesus because the Word says that Jesus Christ is the same yesterday, today and tomorrow.

God's Word also says that heaven and earth shall pass away but His Word shall not pass away.

So healing has to be real for today — just as yesterday — for His Word is for today.

Jesus performed many miracles of healing while He walked here on earth.

The Word teaches us that good health is a priority with God. Healing is an act of grace. Divine health is based on God's Word, common sense, reason and discipline.

Let's look at health through the eyes of God the Father.

Some people say, "Regardless of how I live or how I treat my body, if I get sick God will heal me."

Would you want one of your children to get sick even though you knew you could take the child to the doctor for help? Even though you have the ability to lay hands on the child and pray for healing? Of course not. That would be stupid.

God doesn't want us sick just so He can prove that He can heal us. He wants us to walk in Divine health, free from sickness.

Others say, "Well, God made me sick so I could learn something."

Let's get one thing straight. God never made anyone sick. The devil is the one who puts sickness on people but only if they allow it. He is the one who steals health from people, kills and destroys.

I've fought death and disease and been around sickness for over 20 years and I've yet to see anyone learn anything from it but pain, hurt and financial loss.

Those who have been healed or cured return home hurt in body, hurt in spirit, hurt financially and a tremendous burden to their families. That is not God's plan.

God's plan is for us to walk in Divine health. He did not place your heart in your chest for you to have a heart attack. He put it there to pump life-giving blood, not to be clogged up with plaque, cholesterol and fat.

The only way the devil can put a coronary heart attack on us is for us to allow it. Old Slew Foot gets a lot of credit for things he doesn't deserve.

God will not make you sick and Satan can't make you sick unless you let him. The evil one will give you the opportunity to become ill but you make the choice.

The devil can't touch the Christian's spirit. It belongs to God. But if you allow him into your mind and confess, "I'm getting sick," you will become sick. You then have set a negative spiritual law into effect and thus help Satan make you sick.

The Word says that you are snared by the words of your mouth. It also says that the power of life and death is in the tongue.

There are numerous spiritual laws, both positive and negative, and also natural laws. When we violate these laws we must pay the consequences.

Faith is a spiritual law. By faith we stand against the enemy when he tries to make us sick. Action is also a spiritual law for faith without action is a dead faith.

Love is another spiritual law. It is the opposite of hate. When hate replaces love then you give place to the evil one and he makes you sick.

Remember in the Word where the devil came to Jesus and finding nothing in Him had to leave?

Since we are joint heirs with Christ, if the devil comes and finds nothing in us lacking he can't make us sick. But if we have abused our bodies and given place to the devil, he makes us sick.

If he finds bitterness in the heart, anxiety, stress or fear, then he uses it against us. That's where most ulcers come from.

Bad confession, depression and rebellion against God's Word are also negative spiritual laws which, when violated, lead to sickness.

Let me give you a rule of thumb on positive and negative spiritual laws. If something in your life is good, peaceful and uplifting, then it is of God and positive. If it leads to bitterness, hate or remorse, then it is of Satan and negative.

What are the natural laws which we must obey if we are to have good health?

There is a light switch in my office. If I get up out of my chair, walk to the switch and turn it on, the room is flooded with light. By so doing I put into motion two natural laws. First was the law of physical motion toward the light switch. Second was the physical law of electricity which provided power for the lights. Unless I know those two natural laws, and put them into effect, I would sit in darkness day and night.

Gravity is another natural law. Violate it by jumping off a high place and you will suffer for it.

God has numerous natural laws. What are some of them?

1. Overeating leads to overweight.
2. Lack of exercise causes weakness and poor physical condition.

3. Stress brings about emotional and physical illness.
4. What we eat is what we become.
5. Proper sleep and rest allows the body time to repair itself.
6. A merry heart does good like a medicine but a broken spirit dries the bones.
7. We reap what we sow.

When the spiritual laws function in our lives they greatly influence the natural laws.

For instance, the Word says, ". . . walk in the Spirit, and ye shall not fulfil the lust of the flesh" (Galatians 5:16).

When most people hear the word lust they immediately think of sex. But people also lust after chocolate pie, gravy and gumbo. Remember that Satan used fruit as the very first weapon against man.

Recently I read a report that said the biological deterioration or degeneraton of the human body starts at the age 35 in America. Do you know why? Because we don't take care of ourselves.

Why do Christians feel bad when they wake up in the morning? Because they are carrying around 30 or 40 pounds of extra weight; have high cholesterol and triglyceride levels in their blood; and are out of shape through inactivity. So they are sluggish and tired.

Everything temporal is subject to change. We cannot affect body change just by praying to God to take the fat away from us or to make us exercise. God will never override the will of one of his children if we continue to eat like pigs.

I am confident that if we would follow God's plan and take care of our bodies we could live to be 100 or 120 years old. Medical science has recently made the statement that there is no reason why people shouldn't live from 120 to 140 years.

Have you ever wondered why some Russian peasants live for 125 years? It's simple. They eat the right foods, with plenty of fiber and roughage, work every day until they die and get the rest the body needs to repair itself. Some of those old Russians, even at age 100, continue to walk eight to 10 miles a day to work. We're not saying that everyone should walk eight to 10 miles every day. But proper exercise is necessary for a long, healthful life.

Many Americans, rather than studying why some Russian peasants live so long, had rather play Russian Roulette with their health.

About all the walking most Americans do is from their house to the garage to get into their cars to go to church, the supermarket, school or work.

The prestigious *Wall Street Journal* recently published an intriguing article entitled: ''Ounce of Prevention is Worth a Pound of Cure, or so say proponents of the 'Wellness' Movement.''

''Many companies and their employees have come to feel they should start placing more stress on 'wellness' or preventing disease before there is a need to cure it,'' the *Journal* said. ''Everyone would be better off, proponents of the notion argue, safeguarding health and staving off illness.''

The *Journal* continued: ''The fundamental elements of a wellness program are simple, familiar and beyond controversy: Exercise, sound diet, adequate rest and control of stress. . . .''

"Wellness advocates say that the way modern medicine has been practiced, patients tend to be complacent about their physical condition," the *Journal* said. "They pay obeisance to good health by having an annual physical, and then they return to their normal bad habits."

According to the *Journal* article, practicing wellness is both fun and free. People who follow principles of wellness "are stronger, better-looking, have higher morale, superior bowel movements and more antibodies against disease. They also become wildly popular . . . and get elected to office."

The *Wall Street Journal* article impressed me for I had been saying that to my patients for several years.

Within the framework of God's plan, how is a Christian supposed to feel? Like God feels.

Here's exactly how we are supposed to feel. The Lord's prayer says: " . . . Thy will be done in earth, as it is in heaven" (Matthew 6:10).

There is not one sick person in heaven! God wants us to feel good here on earth.

God never created the heart in the chest to explode into a heart attack or a stroke. He created the joints to function perfectly, not to be swollen and sore because of painful arthritis. He created the gastrointestinal tract to perform perfectly, not to develop ulcers and cancer.

The evil one can't take away the joy we have for it is a fruit of the Spirit. But when we allow him to attack our bodies with sickness then we become unhappy.

We Christians talk a lot about ministry. But

regardless of how spiritual we may feel, if we are sick it is very difficult, if not impossible, to minister out to others.

And, let me repeat, one of the greatest sources of sickness in America today is the eating habits of the people.

One nutritionist suggested that we should be as careful about what we put in our bodies as we are about what we put in our cars.

The majority of us would never dream of putting any bad gas or oil in our cars. They are far too valuable.

But what about the body? It is the most precious, valuable physical possession we have.

God says the body is valuable. Throughout His Word He tells us the value He places on it.

The Word says for us to present our bodies as "a living sacrifice, holy, acceptable unto God . . ." (Romans 12:1). God also says to "glorify God in your body . . ." (I Corinthians 6:20). The Word calls the body "the temple of the Holy Spirit" (I Corinthians 6:19).

God wants us to be in the peak of good health. He created our bodies to work perfectly. And, by following certain biblical principles with obedience and discipline we can feel better and live longer.

Some people I've treated actually get to the point where they think it is normal to feel tired all the time. They have forgotten what it was like to feel good.

Yet, most Christians never stop to ask themselves: "Why don't I feel good?" Many people never give health a second thought until disaster strikes. Then it becomes all important and may be too late.

The Word has a promise for those who honor the Lord in all things. It says: "With long life will I satisfy him . . ." (Psalm 91:16).

But God is not bound to keep that promise if we break his laws regarding physical health and wellness.

God also tells us the Word is "life" to those who find it and "health" to the body.

Listen to the Word when it says: "My son, forget not my law; but let thine heart keep my commandments.

"For length of days, and long life, and peace, shall they add to thee" (Proverbs 3:1-2).

Why can't Christians believe and follow the Word?

One nutritionist said, "Instant satisfaction blocks out any concern about long-term consequences." Or pitted against "delayed effects" the "immediate gratification" is always more important.

People would rather eat the chocolate pie, drink too much coffee, smoke the cigarettes than experience the uncomfortable feeling which accompanies the early stages of abstinence. The "instant gratification" outweighs the long-term dangerous results. They had rather have a magic potion to make the fat fall off than to cleanse their blood vessels. Or, they want to take a pill rather than discipline their eating habits.

I don't like to see Satan rob God's people of health for I know that God wants his people healthy.

Many ministers of the Gospel come to me for help. Often they are overweight, burned out and unable to minister with all their potential strength. I am ever conscious of the fact that if they are well, healthy and live longer they may win thousands more souls to Christ. And, praise God, I'll get some credit for it when the awards are passed out in heaven!

The Word delineates another law commonly called the law of the harvest. It simply explains that we reap what we sow.

We Americans are sowing bad health as teenagers by eating all the junk food, additives, preservatives and becoming too fat. We reap the harvest of those bad eating habits, and general lack of activity, in the 30s and 40s. Remember that heart attacks are epidemic among people in their 40s.

It amazes me that separated, sanctified Christians won't go to the wrong kind of movie, but could care less what they put in their bodies.

Were Christians to take care of themselves the prayer lines in our churches and evangelistic meetings would not be nearly so long. Then, rather than being sick much of the time, God's people could be out helping the lost find Christ and praying for *them* to be healed. Most pastors today have their hands full with sick congregations and thus find it difficult to have enough time to reach out to people living in physical and spiritual hell here on earth.

The Word tells us the body is the temple of God and that if any man "defile the temple" God will destroy him (I Corinthians 3:17).

That willful act — defiling the body — opens the door for the devil to put sickness on us.

Contrariwise, anyone, regardless of age, who begins a life-style of proper diet, adequate exercise and regular relaxation will start feeling better in approximately one week, barring some serious physical illness.

It is impossible to divide tripartite man.

He is spirit, soul and body. It is quite difficult for a

healthy spirit to grow strong when it lives in a sick home.

Our Lord gave thousands of health tips to His chosen people, the Israelites. They were written in the law. These people had no quickie foods, no preservatives or additives, they walked nearly everywhere they went and worked long hours in the fields. Yet God gave them hundreds of rules about how to eat.

Let me repeat there are seven "musts" for good health. They are:

1. Correct eating habits.
2. Correct vitamins and minerals.
3. Adequate sleep.
4. A regular program of exercise.
5. Adequate intake of pure water.
6. A positive outlook on life.
7. A changing of life-style.

Commit these seven "musts" to memory for we will be discussing them in detail in future chapters.

By following these proven principles nearly anyone can develop:

1. More physical energy.
2. A sharper mind.
3. A better memory.
4. Calmness.
5. Coolheadedness.
6. Self-control.
7. Better looks.

Also commit these to memory for they are some of the goals you need to set for yourself as you follow

The Divine Connection toward good health.

There is no substitute for good nutrition. In a later chapter we will deal with the subject in great detail.

Without proper vitamins and minerals the body will never be in optimum health.

Exercise helps the entire body.

It also invigorates the mind and thinking processes. A sedentary life is a great enemy to good health. Exercise also cuts down on stress and helps us handle it much better.

Good sleep and rest gives the body time to repair itself.

Water is the elixir of life.

Samuel Taylor Coleridge, in his famous poem "Rime of the Ancient Mariner" wrote: "Water, water everywhere — but not a drop to drink."

Many Americans have water, water everywhere and don't drink a drop.

Water is a wonderful lubricant which helps the whole body function better. It purifies the system by helping clean out the blood and adequate water helps carry impurities out of the body.

Most women think water is only to be used for cooking and taking baths. We in the practice of medicine see such a large amount of urinary tract involvement, primarily cystitis. Why is that the case? Because women don't drink water.

It's good, it's natural and it's God's solvent. It makes the kidneys work better. Everyone should try it by drinking at least eight full glasses a day.

This seven-pronged approach to good health closely parallels the teaching about health in the scriptures. They are imperative if we want to feel better and live longer.

Let me say that for most of my life I violated all the laws of God as they relate to good health. And, the so-called "good" life nearly killed me. My life-style of overeating, drinking and punishing my body with long work hours and little rest ruined my health. I punished my body so much that I nearly committed long-term suicide.

Bless God He saved and healed me just in time!

During these years since my healing, I have become convinced God would have preferred that I kept my body in good health. His perfect will for me was that I would have remained healthy. His permissive will granted my healing.

CHAPTER 2

Rx for Health

Have you ever taken time to think about how marvelous, how complex, your body is? Most of us take it for granted until something goes wrong.

At the time of conception the sperm of the male penetrates the egg of the female and we are the result of the union of two cells. From this union we become a body comprised of approximately 40 trillion cells.

It was always awesome to deliver a child. The baby's head would sweep under the mother's pelvis brim. I would deliver the head, then the shoulders and finally the buttocks, legs and feet. I would hold the new-born child by its feet, cut the umbilical cord and then thump it to make it breathe.

The child would take a breath, expand its lungs and begin its life here on planet earth.

As I held the babies I often thought, "What a miracle this is!" But never once did I understand that it was a miracle from God.

Do you know something else that amazed me?

During all those years when I delivered countless hundreds of babies while doing OB-GYN, not once did I ever hear a mother give thanks to God for a perfect child. That is not to say no mother ever said it. I just didn't hear it. Many just took the miracle for granted.

That's the way most of us take health — for granted.

We just blunder through life paying little attention to our health. We never miss it until we lose it.

There is a mystique which surrounds the human body. If you don't think so then why are there so many doctor programs on television? People are interested in the human body.

During more than 20 years in medicine I have learned that there are two areas of life which are surrounded by unbelievable superstition — birth and death. People are just naturally interested in where they came from, what they're doing here on earth and where they are going when they die.

A Christian is the strongest person in the world. The problem is the majority of us don't know it.

Christians have been taught all of our lives that we are just poor, no-good sinners saved by grace.

I am not still a sinner saved by grace. I was an old sinner but now I am a child of the living God and joint heir with the Lord Jesus. So I must take care of my body in order to glorify him.

Once while I was traveling in Africa with T.L. Osborn, he said there are only two reasons why Christians fail: (1) The Christian does not know who he is in Christ; and (2) He forgets it.

The body is very important to me as is the health of the body and the mind.

Through the years I have seen people live in physical misery, without happiness and peace. Most of it could have been prevented if they had taken care of themselves.

Without health life can be miserable. I have treated multi-millionaires who were sick. One of them was a 55-year-old man who was dying of emphysema. He once told me he would give all his fortune for one good breath. He destroyed his health accumulating wealth. Then when he got it he had no health to enjoy it.

Divine health is your heritage and inheritance from the Creator. It is a gift of God. But He is not obligated to keep you in health as long as you mistreat your body.

Let me give you some helpful advice on how to take care of yourself.

What about a diet that would help you avoid getting certain forms of cancer?

There is a good, low-risk cancer diet that we all should follow.

Cancer kills many people in the United States.

According to the latest research, the manner in which we cook our food and eat it contributes to 60 percent of the nation's cancer deaths.

When your diet is loaded with fat — such as heavy meat — the liver produces an excessive amount of bile. The bile rushes into the duodenal area to break up the fat. If the bile remains in the colon longer than normal, carcinogenic agents, or cancer-causing agents, can develop.

The bile is not the carcinogenic agent but a high-fat diet having been broken down by the bile can produce the agents.

What is the answer? It's simple. Cut way down on the amount of fat you eat.

There is a second way to avoid certain types of cancer. Add fiber to your diet. It is very important in reducing cancer of the colon.

A high-fiber diet helps counteract the effect of fat on the colon.

What else does fiber do? It adds bulk to the stool and decreases the amount of time the food remains in the bowel thus speeding up elimination. So, if you have a carcinogenic agent passing through the bowel, you can decrease the amount of time it remains there by eating a lot of fiber. You also decrease the chances of cancer.

Where do we get our fiber? One of the best ways is to use one-third cup of Miller's Bran three times a day. It can be sprinkled on cereals but not on toasted cereals. You can also use it in cooking to replace some of your corn meal and flour.

If you don't like bran, use raw cabbage, carrots or apples. They also provide an abundance of fiber. But remember that there are about 135 calories in an apple. Cabbage and carrots have far fewer calories.

Through the years I have seen a lot of bowel cancer. I've operated on them — cut them open, sewed them back — and seen some of them live out the rest of their lives as gastrointestinal cripples.

If you had seen what I've seen, you, too would be interested in preventing cancer.

There is a third ingredient for a low-risk cancer

diet.

Take large doses of vitamin C. It helps protect the gastrointestinal tract against irritants.

We believe that one of the reasons carcinoma of the stomach is less in the United States than in some foreign countries is due to our intake of vitamin C.

For instance, the Japanese don't receive much vitamin C and they have a lot of cases of carcinoma.

Selenium is also an element that reduces the risk of cancer. Research proves it.

Foods rich in selenium include fish, liver, kidneys, onions, garlic, mushrooms, eggs and wheat cereals. You can also buy selenium at the store.

According to a *New York Times* article in March of 1982, scientific concern over what causes cancer is beginning to change.

"For several years there was great concern over cancer-causing substances found in the environment and places where people worked," the *Times* article said. But now scientists are placing less blame on environment and more blame on diet, smoking, alcohol and sexual behavior.

"They blame tobacco for causing 30 percent of the cancer deaths — as does the recent surgeon general's report on smoking and cancer," the *Times* said. "They also suggest that nutritional factors — such as calories, fat, fiber, vitamins, trace elements and other substances that may effect the formation and transport of carcinogens in the body — ultimately may be found of comparable importance."

The article continued: "By comparison, their (researchers) estimates of cancers caused by the products and pollutants of American industry seem

small. Occupational exposures . . . account for only
four percent of American cancer deaths, and pollution in the air, water, food and earth accounts for
even less.''

The *Times* article also noted that sexual and repro-
ductive behavior accounts for some seven percent of
all cancer in the United States.

''The risk of cancer of the cervix, for example, is
increased by having multiple sexual partners. . . .''
The Bible talked about the results of promiscuity centuries ago.

The *Times* quoted one of the researchers as saying:
''The sky is not falling. But the increases (in cancer)
look real, and we had better find out what's causing
them.''

Next I would like for us to discuss the subject of
heart disease for along with cancer, it is one of the
major killers of the people of America today.

On March 15, 1982 the respected *U.S. News* and
World Report magazine ran a cover story entitled
''America's $39 Billion Heart Business.''

Think of it! The nation's bill for treating heart
disease is $39 billion a year!

Heart disease has created a ''booming new industry'' in this country, the magazine pointed out.

U.S. News quoted the following statistics from the
American Heart Association:

1. Americans spend $3.5 billion a year on heart
drugs — compared to $400 million 10 years ago.

2. Yearly costs for hospital and nursing-home care
for heart patients reached $28.7 billion — compared
to $2.2 billion 10 years ago.

3. Coronary-bypass surgery, which was con-

sidered as experimental in the early 1970s, now is reported to be a $3.3-billion-a-year business.

4. Those physicians who treat heart patients receive $7 billion yearly for their services — compared to $1 billion 10 years ago.

The Heart Association says that about 40 million Americans have some form of heart disease and 35 million have high blood pressure. Every year a million people die of heart disorders and strokes, the magazine reported.

"In basic research, scientists are trying to design drugs that would keep the heart disease from developing in the first place . . . working on a synthetic-protein drug that helps the body remove fatty deposits in the blood," the magazine said.

This all just astounds me!

Through the years I've sent my heart patients to the great hospitals of the nation for bypass surgery and other treatment. The skilled surgeons performed the surgery, the patient improved remarkably, then was dismissed from the hospital and sent home — on the same diet that caused the heart trouble in the first place.

Little or no information was given the heart patient on what caused the problems. Nothing about diet, triglycerides, fat, cholesterol, exercise, stress, being overweight, smoking, rest — nothing.

Now scientists are trying to find a synthetic medicine that will reduce fatty substances in the blood. Why put them there in the first place? Proper diet will keep them out.

Let me give you Dr. Whitaker's plan for a healthy heart:

1. Eat right. Balance your meals. Take proper vitamins, minerals and trace elements.
2. Lose weight. Don't go even a pound over what you should weigh.
3. Quit smoking. It'll kill you.
4. Exercise. Learn what is best for you. Then stick to it.
5. Get plenty of rest. Learn how to sleep well at night.
6. Conquer stress. Exercise helps. Learn to deal with stressful situations. Develop a hobby or other interest besides your work.
7. See your doctor regularly.
8. Cut down on fat, sugar and white flour. They are poison.

Although this lifetime regimen may seem a high mountain to climb, isn't it better than open-heart surgery, heart attacks and strokes?

There is another dividend. You will feel better and live longer. And life will be so much more enjoyable.

CHAPTER 3

Freedom From Sickness

We know it is God's perfect will for us to "be in health."

Then why are so many Christians sick?

There are numerous reasons.

First, Satan can touch a Christian's mind and body but only if the Christian cooperates and allows it.

Jesus called Satan a thief who came to kill, rob and destroy. He would like to kill or destroy every Christian and would were he not restrained by a loving God.

Once we become Christians the evil one bombards our minds and bodies with every potential disease imaginable.

Your soul, or mind, is made up of all the experiences you have had throughout your life.

It is important that you not give place to the devil. If you do, if you cooperate with him, he afflicts your body and mind.

Therefore, prevention — or wellness — is essential if we are to remain free from illness.

Your body was created out of the earth's dust. It belongs to the planet. Therefore, it is subject to the laws of nature. Violate those laws and you give place to the devil to make you sick.

When you die your body will return to dust or to the planet from which it was created. Of course the spirit will go to be with God for all eternity.

The body is subject to all the rules of this planet as well as to God's natural laws.

For instance, if you step out in front of a speeding car, you must pay the price. That car will kill you for you are subject to the laws of force and thrust.

If you step off a 10-story building, you will soon discover you are subject to the natural laws of gravity as you fall.

Likewise, your body is subject to Divine health laws. Break them and you come to the bitter end — sickness.

The Word explains in Matthew 4:14-32 that there are five ways Satan attacks us. They include:

1. Affliction — making us sick.
2. Persecution — for the Word's sake.
3. Lust — wanting others or other things.
4. Cares — worry over circumstances.
5. Deceitfulness — over riches.

Note that three of the five — affliction, lust and cares — all relate to the mind and body.

The Apostle Paul carefully spelled out that concept when he warned the members of the early church about disobeying the laws of God.

He said: "Whose end is destruction, whose God is their belly, and whose glory is in their shame" (Philippians 3:19).

The subject of food is a recurring theme throughout the scriptures.

Satan used the lust for food to take Esau's birthright away from him. Esau was so ravenous for food he was willing to give up everything — just for a mess of pottage. Pottage was a mixture of beans, peas and lentils or eatable seeds. Boiled with oil and garlic it made a delightful meal.

After Jesus fasted 40 days and nights, the evil one appeared to him and tempted him. What was the object of the temptation? Bread.

Jesus, though hungry, turned him back by declaring there are more important things in life than food.

As I have traveled throughout the world I've seen hoards of hungry people. Millions of them go to bed hungry at night hoping they will be able to find enough food to make it through the next day.

However, there are probably as many as 60 million Americans who go to bed at night and pray they will have the willpower not to over-indulge in food the next day.

Most of them do have stomach distress during the night and that's the reason sales are booming for the companies which manufacture anti-acids.

God recently revealed to me that millions of Christians are dying needlessly because of the food they eat.

Good nutrition, or good eating habits, helps us cooperate with God's plan for Divine health. It lets us stand against the evil one who would make us sick.

A lot of Christians say, "Well, I'll just bless the food and ask God to protect me." Then they gorge on all the wrong things.

Or, some Christians say, "I'll go ahead and eat what I want and smoke my cigarettes and if I get sick God will heal me."

Because of his goodness and love God does heal many of them.

But what about the ones who don't get healed?

I'm convinced God's perfect plan is for us to stay healthy. God's permissive will is for us to lay hands on the sick and see them healed.

Let's take a look at some dangerous foods and the illnesses they can cause.

Sugar

Sugar is like poison to the body.

It can cause heart disease, high blood pressure, cancer, fatigue, anxiety, hyperactivity, ulcers, diseases of the colon, allergies, diabetes, hypoglycemia, migraine headaches and behavioral disorders, including schizophrenia, the most dreaded of all mental illnesses, obesity and high blood pressure.

Why is sugar such a problem? It is usually in foods that contain empty calories — foods that provide filler but little food value. So people who eat a lot of food with a high content of sugar may feel full all the time but actually are undernourished.

Sugar causes the triglyceride level in the blood to increase and can cause heart disease.

People who eat some sugar crave more. Before the craving is satisfied the person has eaten far too much.

That kind of diet usually includes cancer-causing additives, dyes, food coloring and preservatives.

Each American consumes about 120-130 pounds of white sugar each year. We eat much of it in junk foods.

Sugar robs the body of the B-complex vitamins — just wipes them out. They are essential in breaking down carbohydrates, which are necessary for energy and appetite control.

A lack of the B-complexes can lead to nerve disorders, heart palpitations, heart disease, increased cholesterol. Why are the B-complexes so important? They help clear the slug out of the blood vessels.

The really bad thing about white sugar is that it takes the place of the good food you should be eating and has absolutely no nutritional value. Sugar is just a thief.

It also causes cavities in your teeth and in some cases contributes to emotional problems.

Sugar steals thiamin from the body. A deficiency in thiamin can cause anxiety, nervousness, poor memory, confusion and forgetfulness. Such a deficiency also can result in hyperactivity in children and hypoglycemia in adults.

That's what sugar can do for you.

My patients often say: "I don't eat 130 pounds of sugar a year."

My reply is: "You probably don't eat that much out of a sugar bowl."

However, there is a lot of hidden sugar. It can be found in bread, canned goods, salad dressings, various mixes, condensed juices and other foods.

Read the labels. Remember that OSE added to the

end of a word usually means a product of sugar.

People often ask me what I use to sweeten my food. I use a little honey that has not been refined. But don't use the honey that is real clear for it has been subject to filtration, having been through filters under approximately 400 pounds of pressure. That breaks down and takes out most of the vitamins and minerals that are present in the natural honey. The natural honey that is a little cloudy is the best.

Remember that junk foods contain a lot of the simple carbohydrates — that's why they are called junk.

Simple carbohydrates are also in abundance in white bread, white rice, noodles, macaroni, spaghetti, canned fruits, potato chips, muffins, cakes, cookies, pies, pretzels, candy bars, chocolate, jams and jellies, ice cream and soft drinks.

Here is the content of hidden sugars in certain foods.

Canned fruit has about four teaspoons of sugar per half cup. Two ounces of chocolate bar has eight teaspoons. One glazed donut has six. Twelve ounces of soft drink, eight. One piece of chocolate cake, 15. A banana split, 25. One milk shake, 25.

Have you ever noticed when you drink a Coke and spill some of it on your hand that it is sticky? That's because it's loaded with sugar.

We must learn to replace the junk foods with fresh fruit and vegetables, and grains and wheat bread that hasn't been processed. We also should learn to eat beans, peas, poultry and the cheaper cuts of beef. We Americans are not accustomed to eating right. That's why we don't feel good. That's why we die young. That's why we have heart disease, diabetes and cancer. That's why we're fat and lazy.

The American people should be sick and tired of being sick and tired. Most Americans go to the doctor for a lot of expensive tests. The doctor says he can't find anything wrong. Then you wonder if you are crazy.

No. The problem is that your whole body is nutritionally out of balance. Your vitamins — particularly the B-complex vitamins — are out of order. And sugar usually is the culprit.

Do you know what happens to sugar cane once it is cut? It is taken through 14 processes. Thus, all the enzymes, protein, B-complex vitamins and minerals are taken out of it. What remains? White sugar which is basically worthless. The by-product of all that processing of sugar is black strap molasses.

Let me give you a personal word about white sugar.

I have some bad teeth because of all the white sugar I ate as a child. Then while playing football several of my teeth were knocked loose.

Had I known then what I know now, my life could have been spared several diseases which attacked me, including heart disease, high blood pressure, pancreatitis and bad teeth.

God healed me of the pancreatitis through a miracle. But I have corrected my diet. God helped me make that correction but never forced me to do it. That was an act of choice.

Now my blood pressure and EKG are normal and I feel great all the time!

Due to all the warning signs you would think people would quit eating junk foods. But Americans, and particularly children, are eating more junk than ever before.

The next time you visit a school take a look at the children. You will be amazed that so many of them are fat. They are eating too much junk food.

A friend of mine designs fashion jeans for a firm in New York City. She said recently that the firm designed a new line of women's fashion jeans because the rear ends of the American women had expanded so much that a new line was required.

What about smoking?

Again there are natural laws. If broken, the penalty must be paid.

There are three good reasons to quit smoking: HEART ATTACK, LUNG CANCER and EMPHYSEMA.

There are several other good reasons to quit smoking:

1. It saps a person's energy.
2. It causes shortness of breath.
3. It makes one smell bad.
4. It can cause the eyesight to deteriorate.
5. It can cause the complexion to be bad.
6. It causes the capillaries, veins and arteries to constrict.
7. It causes the skin to age.
8. A female who is pregnant and smokes is doing a disservice to the unborn child.
9. It hurts the children who must smell the smoke.
10. It dishonors the "temple" of God and therefore dishonors God.

Junk food dishonors God and causes harm to the body.

You won't find any reference to junk food in the scriptures except in the Proverbs where it talks about putting away from yourself the perversion of food. One translation renders the word "perversion" as "deceitful." This simply means that some food deceives the body.

It also means that some food looks good and tastes good but is not good for you.

Like pork.

The Word says: "And the swine . . . is unclean to you," (Leviticus 11:7).

When the great Prophet Isaiah cried out against the rebellion of the Jews, he said that one of their acts of rebellion toward God was eating swine's flesh (Isaiah 65:4).

Do you remember when Jesus cast out the demons from the men in the tombs? The demons were so numerous they went into a large herd of pigs. The pig-keepers were so scared they high-tailed it to the city for help.

What were those Jews doing keeping pigs around? Probably because they enjoyed eating pork — like most Americans.

Don't eat pork. It has too much fat, thus cholesterol, and causes heart disease and other illnesses.

Wouldn't you agree that it is better to prevent disease than to go through diagnosis and treatment and weeks, months or even years of sickness?

Wellness and prevention are the best money bargains available.

Ordinarily your insurance will pay about 80 percent of your costs at a preventive medicine clinic. Therefore, the average person can afford it. And it will be the best money you have ever spent.

If you can stay out of the hospital, and particularly out of the intensive care unit or coronary care unit, think of how much money you can save.

But there is more — you just feel so much better and enjoy life more.

Let's take a look at psychosomatic illnesses.

About 80 percent of all hospital beds are occupied by people with some form of mental illness.

One of the major causes is worry. Did you know that "worry" and "drunkenness" are mentioned in the same sentence in the Word?

God wants you to be happy but that is impossible if you are filled with worry for it causes your whole body to get out of kilter.

Worry is a sin and is very destructive.

When you worry it causes your body to suffer.

But not everyone who is diagnosed as neurotic is in fact neurotic. What they need is a good nutritional evaluation.

Do you know that there are a lot of people in mental institutions who really don't belong there? They are deficient in enzymes, co-enzymes, vitamins, minerals and supplements.

Nutrition can help all forms of mental illness except manic depression.

Extensive research had concluded that diet is one of the basic causes of hyperactivity in children. This hyperactivity can lead to worry and mental illness. Proper nutrition can control the problem.

Jesus himself told us there is never any cause to

worry. He said the Father takes care of us when we first seek the kingdom of God.

Stress is a real problem in our society today, and why not? If you watch the 6:00 o'clock news what do you see? Rape, muggings, killings, car wrecks, plane crashes, child abuse, corruption in government and corporate theft.

No wonder people have so much stress.

People worry about a nuclear attack, threat of financial hard times, threat of loss of health, fear of growing old, problems in society, difficulties with wayward children — and it all creates stress.

Just remember that all is well in heaven and there is no depression there. People are just moving too fast and worrying too much. We need to learn to slow down.

During the first 15 years I was in medicine I hardly ever looked up. In one three-year period I only took one weekend off for relaxation. My financial statement was fine but I was spiritually, mentally and physically bankrupt.

There is much more to life than running at a high speed in the fast lane trying to make a dollar.

We need to learn to smell the flowers, see the trees, watch the ocean and enjoy little children.

Those simple disciplines will do much to alleviate stress.

The Word says: "Trust in the Lord with all thine heart; and lean not unto thine own understanding.

"In all thy ways acknowledge him and he shall direct thy paths" (Proverbs 3:5-6).

There are some other ways to solve the stress problem in your life.

1. Learn to know and rely on Jesus.
2. Meditate and trust His Word.
3. Get some good exercise.
4. Develop a hobby or some interest to get your mind off your problems.
5. Get plenty of rest.
6. Take your family swimming or on a picnic or for a walk in the woods.

You can experience a miraculous victory over stress.

Caffeine can also be a hazard to your health. Coffee, tea and certain colas contain caffeine in substantial amounts.

Were caffeine to be introduced on the market today the Federal Drug Administration would require a prescription for you to buy it. The drug is very potent and addictive.

Caffeine can actually kill. Massive doses fed to laboratory animals produced cancer and heart disease. Too much caffeine also damages the liver which produces important digestive juices necessary for good health.

It was most difficult for me to give up coffee. We always kept a pot of coffee in the emergency room, one in surgery, one in the lab and one on each floor of the hospital. I drank about three pots of coffee a day.

Caffeine consumed by pregnant women can have adverse effects on the unborn baby. Tests have shown that some such babies are born with less muscle tone and are less active than normal.

Caffeine causes some people's hearts to flutter or run rapidly.

The heart has four chambers — two atria on the

top, two ventricles on the bottom. When some people drink too much coffee the atrium flutters causing shortness of breath and dizziness because the brain is not getting enough oxygen.

God healed me of that very illness and now I don't have to worry about it.

But why should I give place to the devil by going back to drinking three pots of coffee a day?

I now drink two cups a day, one-half cup at a time. I fill my cup half with coffee, half with water.

My mind thinks I'm getting a good cup of coffee four times a day.

Listen to your body. It will tell you when you are drinking too much coffee, tea or colas, thus taking in too much caffeine.

Some people have said, "My goodness, Dr. Whitaker, you're strict."

"Not really, I just want the body of Christ to be in good health and enjoy life."

The key words are knowledge and discipline. I can supply the knowledge but you must furnish the discipline.

CHAPTER 4

A Look at the Body

Let's take a look at the anatomy or the structural makeup of the body so that we may better understand the meaning of total health.

There is an old axiom which says: "We are what we eat." Let me expand on that and say the result of what we become physically is also based on what and how we eat.

The food we take into our bodies — and how it is digested — has more effect on the way we feel and the way our body functions than anything else we do.

What do we do day after day, week after week, month after month and year after year? We eat. So, how we manage those large quantities of food determines our eventual state of health.

Proper digestion of food begins in the mouth. Digestion simply means the breaking down of food products so they can be utilized for the whole body.

Most Americans are in such a hurry that they make two initial mistakes which lead to improper digestion — right in the mouth.

First, they do not chew the food properly and just gulp it down or wash it down with coffee, tea, or water. Thus the initial chemical reaction on the food is retarded as it speeds through the mouth on its way to the stomach. The food does not remain in the mouth long enough for the first stage of the digestive process to take place.

Second, large numbers of people do not relax when they eat. This further impedes good digestion.

Under these circumstances, proper digestion never has a chance. The result is that the body does not receive the full value from the food, and, because of improper digestion in the mouth, all kinds of stomach discomfort may result.

The reason anti-acids are leading sellers in the United States is due to improper digestion due to improper eating habits due to improper chewing and lack of chewing or fast eating.

Here's an idea that can help you solve the digestion problem. While you eat, sit on your right hand and eat with your left hand. That will slow you down.

Some anti-acids do provide temporary relief from stomach discomfort but give no long-range answers to proper nutrition and digestion.

It amazes me that some people — particularly women — eat while standing up. Proper relaxation, which enhances good digestion, is difficult to achieve while standing up and eating.

Housewives do all their tasting standing up, then can't imagine why they have upset stomachs. Many of them are seldom hungry when they go to the table to eat the meal they prepared.

One woman who was rather dangerously over-weight came to my office to begin a nutrition and weight-control program. One of the questions I routinely ask is: "How much do you eat at suppertime?"

"Oh, Dr. Whitaker, I don't eat much of anything at supper," she replied.

Then I discovered the reason why she was over-weight — she had tasted the food.

Let me admit that if I had to spend several hours a day in the kitchen I would probably weigh 300 pounds. I once weighed 272 pounds. I'm six feet four inches tall — but 272 was a bit much.

So I know how awful it feels to be fat, with my clothes bulging out in all the wrong places. I know how it feels to be unable to comfortably bend over and pull up my boots.

I used to walk into a room full of people and find the fattest person there. I would amble over toward that person and stand real close so I wouldn't be the biggest one at the party. At times it was hard to find someone bigger than I.

The road to becoming fat starts in the mouth with wrong eating habits which lead to improper digestion.

The study of the anatomy of the body also teaches us that the food passes from the mouth through the esophagus. The esophagus, a muscular tube, extends from the pharynx to the stomach and usually is about nine inches long.

We Americans in general know very little about what takes place in the stomach as it relates to digestion and good health. We just stuff it full of loads of food and hope for the best, hope for a feeling of comfort and well being. Often the result is just the opposite.

Our traditional eating habits amaze me. We start with a salad and then take liquid. Next we eat protein and starches and wash them down. Then comes dessert and finally coffee or some other liquid.

That is the wrong way to eat.

To achieve the best digestive results we should always eat our protein first. The Europeans have done that for decades. And, their incidence of stomach disorders is far less than ours. They also have less stomach cancer.

The reason we should eat proteins first is very simple. We have hydrochloric acid — a gastric juice — in the stomach. We also have renin and pepsin — enzymes which break down protein and aid digestion. We have these enzymes in large amounts in the stomach but to a large extent they are only effective in breaking down protein.

After we eat the meat or other protein food we then eat vegetables. After the vegetables we eat salad. After salad, dessert, ·which we almost always should avoid. Except, perhaps, for a little fruit and cheese.

When we eat the protein first the major portion of the hydrocholoric acid begins breaking it down thus leading to nature's plan for good digestion.

The digestion of carbohydrates really begins in the mouth, the result of interaction of the food with certain glands located there. These glands produce enzymes which serve as a catalyst for properly breaking down carbohydrates.

Although it is a good idea to chew meat well, no actual digestion of meat takes place until it reaches the stomach.

Sometime ago I was on an ocean cruise with Vicki Jamison and a number of other women.

During a meal one of the ladies turned blue in the face and fell over, right into her food.

Everyone around her thought she had a heart attack. But I sensed she had some food lodged in her throat. We helped dislodge the food and after a few minutes she was all right. She, like many others, just got in too big a hurry and ate too fast — I mean really super fast.

The stomach is an organ that is used primarily for digestion. But it also stores food for a period of time. After digestion of a regular meal the carbohydrates are the first foods to empty out of the stomach. But it takes six to eight hours for meat to digest so it is temporarily stored there.

Let me give you another helpful hint for good digestion and hence good health. Never drink any liquids with your meals.

Does that surprise you? I'm sure it does. It is a great American tradition to guzzle water or some other liquid with everything we eat. No one, and I mean no one, wants to suffer through a meal without water or some other drink. It just adds a feeling of comfort, at least we think.

It is wise not to drink anything 30 minutes before a meal and two hours after a meal.

There are two important reasons for abstaining from liquids with meals.

First, the enzymes and hydrochloric acid help digest the food in the stomach. This is a beautiful part of the creative act of God. Unless we pour fluid down on top of the food.

The fluid dilutes the hydrochloric acid and enzymes and upsets the acid content in the stomach. Thus we decrease their effectiveness and digestion slows down to a crawl — depending on the amount of liquid you drink.

I realize such a concept is hard to accept, particularly if you were like me and used to enjoy large quantities of iced tea with the noon and evening meals.

Second, fluids just don't mix with the acid and enzymes which are working so valiantly to digest the food.

Let me give you an example of how it works.

Have you ever tried to mix oil and water? It doesn't work.

While meat is being digested it releases grease and oil. It mixes well with the hydrochloric acid and enzymes. But when you put water on top of the oil it refuses to mix. That is why you often have a feeling of bloating or uncomfortable fullness.

It may be a difficult discipline to master, but I will guarantee that if you avoid liquids with all meals, within two weeks the bulk of your gastrointestinal complaints will disappear like magic.

Of course it's not magic. It's just eating in compliance with the wonderful way God created our magnificent bodies. The body really works like a charm if we don't abuse it.

Another good health tip on eating and digestion is that we should never eat anything after 7:00 p.m.

That's really hard on us Christians!

I have a theory on why so many Christians overeat. First, we don't smoke — it causes lung cancer. Second, we don't drink — it makes fools out of us.

Third, we don't carouse or party — that's the wrong crowd. So, bless God, we eat and eat and eat.

Have you ever been to a church party or dinner-on-the-grounds where there wasn't any fattening food? Have you ever been to such a church function where they served health food? No. All the mamas bring their best recipes and they are all fattening, usually eaten after 7:00, and we love it.

Even our Sunday School classes often have donuts or cinnamon rolls and coffee around when we fellowship prior to class time. No wonder half of the people get sleepy during the morning sermon which follows.

In order to achieve good health we must be brutally frank with ourselves about our eating habits. We must establish priorities. We can either eat right, have good health and live longer, or eat junk, get sick and die long before our time.

Let me give you another reason why we shouldn't eat anything after 7 p.m.

You will recall that I said that meats remain in the stomach about six to eight hours. Do you know what your body is supposed to be doing when you are asleep? It should be resting. To achieve proper rest the stomach and gastrointestinal tract should be empty so there will be no excessive amount of work on the heart during the sleeping hours.

Do you realize that when the stomach is full a lot of blood is routed from the heart and must go to the stomach to aid digestion? That is why a lot of heart patients have angina and sub sternal pain after a heavy meal. Often patients will come to my office with chest pains. I always ask them when their pains began and many times they will say it was after they ate a meal.

How does this happen? A heavy meal in the stomach causes a shift of circulation to various degrees due to the increased need for blood in the greater and lesser curvature of the stomach to aid in digestion and metabolism. Many times the shift of circulation will cause a decreased amount of flow to be available to the walls of the heart. This can cause chest pains.

So, when you go to bed, your stomach is supposed to be relatively empty. The heart should be pumping just enough blood necessary to keep up the basal metabolism. However, if you go to bed with a stomach full of food that food must be digested.

Under those circumstances you are probably in for a rough night. You lie there, probably toss and turn and if indigestion attacks, you get up and take an anti-acid so you can get to sleep. At 5 a.m. you get up and say to yourself, "I'm just as tired as I was when I went to bed."

Sure you are tired. You don't feel like you got any sleep at all. You should be tired. While you were asleep your body was still working trying to digest all the food you ate just before going to bed.

The Lord has blessed me with the privilege of speaking at Full Gospel Businessmen's meetings all over the world. These dear Christian brothers must have some unwritten rule that they always feed a speaker a heavy meal after each meeting.

Now when they take me to eat after a meeting I just sit there and smile at them but I feel great most of the time. And one of the reasons is because I don't eat a lot of food late at night.

America is the only country where I travel where people can get anything they want to eat day or night.

You won't find that same situation in Europe, unless you are in an area where there are large numbers of Americans. Restaurant owners in those areas stay open all night — as long as the Americans spend bucks on something to eat.

But if you were to travel with me in the rural areas of many foreign lands you would discover that the people never eat past about 6:00 p.m. They have learned a very important health principle on how to take care of themselves. They don't load up their stomachs with food just before going to bed.

There is yet another very important reason why we should not eat after 7:00 p.m.

While we are lying down the gastrointestinal contents in the stomach push up against the diaphragm, which is a muscle that separates the abdominal and thoracic cavities and functions in inhaling and exhaling. The stomach pushes up against the diaphragm and causes an enlargement where the esophagus comes through the orifice into the diaphragm. This situation can cause hiatal hernias which ordinarily are caused by abdominal pressure.

When I encourage you not to eat after 7:00 p.m. I'm not just being mean or trying to deprive you from one of your great pleasures in life. But because it is a proven principle for good health.

It is so simple to take care of ourselves that many of us overlook it.

After four or five hours of digestion in the stomach some of the food passes down through the duodenal area or the first part of the small intestine. In this area there is a duct-like system that comes from the pancreas, and secretes some of the most powerful enzymes in the body, including amylase, trypsin and lipase.

It was those very enzymes which almost killed me in 1975.

My pancreas was completely destroyed because I had been living the "good" life — living to eat instead of eating to live. I was eating too much, drinking too much and weighed 272 pounds. My whole life was totally out of whack.

Because of my life-style the amylase and trypsin started eating up my pancreas. The enzymes began digesting my body instead of my food in my duodenal area. My body was literally being eaten alive by these powerful enzymes and the pain was unbearable.

So the food goes into the small intestine from where additional digestion and then absorption takes place. These enzymes from the pancreas join hydrocholoric acid, bile and limited enzymes produced in the small intestine.

This digestion and absorption takes place over a period of several days and that is why an eating program which includes adequate fiber is so very important. There are numerous studies now being conducted which show a great deal of cancer, particularly cancer of the colon, is related to diet. We also know that heart disease is closely related to diet.

We must be doing something wrong in the way we are eating.

You can never fully understand the seriousness of this matter until you have cared for a person dying of cancer. If you have never gone in and out of a patient's room day after day and watched him as he agonizes in pain. If you have never put him on chemotherapy or done surgery — then stand by and watch him waste away to nothing. Cancer is such a terrible disease.

One of the most difficult tasks in my profession is when I must tell a patient he has incurable cancer. I may even say that through surgery we may cut out the malignancy and I feel we can get it all out and he will survive. But he seldom ever hears anything beyond the word "cancer." Even after surgery and therapy and the person is theoretically cured, he continues to have a terrible horror of the dread disease. This is the reason I know it is much better to prevent cancer than to treat it.

Medical research has determined that those whose diets include a high fiber content have less cancer of the colon than those with a low fiber content.

I can inform you which foods appear to cause cancer of the large bowel and the foods that help prevent it. But I can't eat the food for you, that's your choice. We can prevent a lot of cancer through proper eating and in another chapter I am going to show you how.

God has endowed you with a power of choice concerning how you discipline your eating habits.

Our Lord spelled it out for us in the Old Testament when he wrote: "Behold, I set before you this day a blessing and a curse;

"A blessing, if ye obey the commandments of the Lord your God . . .

"And a curse if ye will not obey the commandments . . ." (Deuteronomy 11:26-28).

The Lord said, "Choose."

Jesus is the captain of our salvation. He has given us the power to lay hands on the sick for their healing and power to cast out demons. He has also given us the responsibility to determine what we stuff into our mouths.

He will never force good eating habits on us. He has turned over to us our choices — what we read, what we watch on television, what we eat.

The Word says: "Therefore to him that knoweth to do good, and doeth it not, to him it is sin" (James 4:17). Proper eating glorifies God because we feel better and live longer. It is an awesome responsibility.

Let's take a look at absorption.

Absorption is the process whereby the food-like material is absorbed from the gastrointestinal tract by little pouches called villi. There are millions of these pouches in the wall of the small intestine.

As the food is broken down by the gastric juices and enzymes it is absorbed into the bloodstream and carried into the body to be used by various organs.

From the small intestine the food which was not absorbed into the bloodstream passes into the large bowel and on to the rectum where the waste is discharged from the body.

Now let's go through the entire process so you can know exactly what happens when you take a bit of food.

When the food enters your mouth the most complex chemical process in the world goes into action. It is called metabolism.

Metabolism

Metabolism is the process and rate by which the cells in the body connect digested material. Here is a simple outline of how it works:

1. Food is taken into the mouth.
2. It passes through the esophagus.
3. It enters the stomach.
4. It is acted on by enzymes and hydrochloric acid.
5. Liquids start passing out of the stomach in 15 to 30 minutes.
6. Carbohydrates remain in the stomach for two or three hours.
7. Fats and meats remain in the stomach six to eight hours.
8. Carbohydrates digestion begins in the mouth.
9. Meats are largely digested in the stomach.
10. Absorption into the blood stream takes place in the small intestine.
11. After absorption the waste material called fecal material is transported to the large intestine. However, most of the absorption and digestion has already taken place in the small intestines. The function of the colon is to move the waste product from digestion and absorption to the sigmoid colon through the rectum.

CHAPTER 5

Eat Right and Like It

During the years of the practice of orthomolecular and preventive medicine I have discovered that most people have very little knowledge about nutrition.

Therefore, let's make a quick study of the subject since understanding nutrition is essential to good health.

Nutrition is the relationship of food to the health of the body.

We are facing a great nutrition crisis in America and it has created a critical national health problem.

My present practice of medicine is primarily related to the body of Christ or Christian people. And of the hundreds of them I have examined about 95 percent of them are in bad health. Their ailments may not cause them to die tomorrow or the next day but they have health problems which keep them from feeling good. For them, nutrition is a prevailing problem.

Do you know what the first symptom is in about 50 percent of all coronary heart attacks? Sudden death.

Death is nature's way of slowing a person down — to a dead stop.

You have heard people say, "He was healthy as a horse and just fell over dead."

That's not true for he really wasn't healthy. The problem had been developing over a period of years. Eating habits, being overweight, smoking, drinking, lack of exercise — all were contributing factors.

The Senate Select Committee On Nutrition and Human Needs conducted a study which reported that six of the 10 major causes of death are closely related to diet. The study included heart disease, stroke, cancer and many other causes of death.

My evaluation of that report convinces me that six out of the 10 major causes of death can be prevented through proper diet — if we will change our eating habits and begin to understand nutrition.

Except for Finland, the United States leads the world in cardiovascular accidents. The reason is that Finland is the only nation on earth that eats more animal fat than we Americans.

This is a nation made up of fat, lazy people who no longer eat properly and get very little exercise.

For 15 years I have given medical examinations for children entering the Head Start Program. During the past four years I kept records on the children.

Our objective in the examinations was to determine if the children were anemic. We did this by taking blood samples and testing them in the laboratory.

We discovered that the number of children tested

who were anemic increased 35 percent — in just four years. Those who were fat jumped 38 percent in that same period.

What does that tell me?

It says that Mama is feeding junk to junior.

Mama may not have time for junior so she puts some food in his mouth to keep him quiet. She feeds junior a donut and says, "Now, shut up junior." Or, she gives him a Coke to drink and says, "Drink it and be quiet. Nice junior."

So junior gets sick and junior's teeth fall out. Mama wonders, "How could that have happened? I gave junior everything he wanted." That was the problem. It begins in childhood and continues into adulthood.

We must have proper nutrition to feel better and live longer. So let's set up some dietary goals.

These are very important, yet minimal goals. If you were to cut down as far as I would like you would all squeal.

1. Increase to 50 percent your consumption of complex carbohydrates obtained from vegetables, grains and legumes.
2. Reduce your consumption of fat to about 30 percent of your diet.
3. Reduce your consumption of saturated fats to about 10 percent.
4. Reduce your cholesterol consumption to about 300 milligrams per day.
5. Omit, as far as possible, all refined sugars.
6. Reduce the amount of salt you eat by 80 percent.
7. Reduce the amount of animal protein that you eat.

How do we accomplish all this? By taking a new look at food and by applying good nutrition to meet our physical needs.

Each of us has the same basic needs. We all need good food, vitamins and minerals. But not one of us needs them in the same ratio because each of us has a different biochemical structure.

Our biochemical patterns of need are like fingerprints, each one is different.

We all must have the six essential nutrients. They include the following:

1. Carbohydrates.
2. Proteins.
3. Fats.
4. Minerals.
5. Vitamins.
6. Water.

For nothing in life affects our bodies as much as the food we eat.

We Christians should be acutely aware of the importance of food.

The Apostle Paul issued a word of caution when he wrote; "I beseech you therefore, brethren, by the mercies of God, that ye present your bodies a living sacrifice, holy, acceptable unto God, which is your reasonable (spiritual) service" (Romans 12:1).

But how can we present our bodies as a holy, acceptable and living sacrifice if we slowly commit suicide by eating junk and fattening foods?

Obviously we can't. So there is a spiritual dimension to good health.

Think about it. Day after day, week after week,

month after month we, by choice, feed our bodies. If we choose to take in good, nutritional food then we will be healthy. But if we choose fattening, junk food then our bodies will develop problems.

Now let's take a closer look at three of these essential nutrients.

Carbohydrates

Carbohydrates are the chief source of energy for the cells of the body. These include sugars, starches and cellulose.

When we say that carbohydrates provide food energy for the cells we are talking about all the body functions of cells, including those in the brain, muscles and cardiovascular system.

When we move or exercise our muscles we break down carbohydrates.

We get complex carbohydrates — the good ones — from starches, grains and vegetables. Simple carbohydrates — the bad ones — come from sugar, white flour and white rice. We also get simple carbohydrates from processed grains.

Fruit is made up of simple carbohydrates but has not been processed. Thus it is a good source of simple carbohydrates.

Most people are confused about the relationship of energy to simple and complex carbohydrates. Some, needing a quick sugar fix, will eat a candy bar and soon will feel much more energetic. But it lasts only about 15 minutes. Then they eat another for more energy.

Energy derived from complex carbohydrates is quite different. We continue to receive energy from them for eight to 10 hours. They also help us digest and assimilate our food and regulate fat and protein metabolism.

Simple carbohydrates poison the body over a long period of time. Not immediately but slowly.

Those who continually stuff themselves on candy, cake, pastries, colas, malts, shakes and sundaes often experience energy lag. But those who receive their carbohydrates from starches, grain, fruits and vegetables have more energy and feel much better longer. They are not always sleepy, tired and run down.

When we eat the refined carbodydrates — with a high sugar content — they tend to decrease the amounts of vitamins and minerals in the system, particularly the B-complex vitamins. That alone is enough to make a person feel bad.

Refined carbohydrates also are like fillers in our food content. They take up space in our stomachs which should be reserved for nutritious food.

They also add extra, unneeded pounds, and increase cholesterol and triglyceride levels in our blood. That makes them extremely dangerous.

We know that too much cholesterol causes arteriosclerosis or the thickening and hardening of the arteries. Ordinarily this illness affects the elderly but recent studies indicate there is no need for anyone — even the elderly — to have hardening of the arteries. This condition simply results from bad eating patterns and the elderly just resign themselves to it.

Therefore if we want to feel better and live longer we must severely limit our intake of the simple carbohydrates and increase the complex ones.

Proteins

Proteins supply the nutrients which are major sources for building up our bodies. Proteins contain amino acids made up of carbon, hydrogen, nitrogen, oxygen and usually sulphur which are essential for strong bodies.

Next to water, protein is the most plentiful substance in the body. Common sense tells us we need an ample supply of it.

Protein is essential for all the tissue of the body and particularly necessary for hair, eyes and teeth. It helps us maintain good health.

Some people have a common misconception that meat is the only source of protein. That is incorrect. Dairy products and eggs also are good sources. However, a person with high cholesterol should limit the number of eggs eaten to about two each week.

Other good sources of protein are fish, brewer's yeast, seeds and grains, soybeans, natural brown rice, rye, oats, millet, wheat and beans.

Plant foods will supply us with adequate protein. But they are not complete and must be interchanged. By interchange I mean certain kinds of protein vegetables must be eaten together in order to receive a proper balance.

Plant proteins, or non-animal proteins, are the very best because they provide bulk, contain no cholesterol, don't elevate triglycerides or cholesterol and are generally so much healthier. They are also much more economical than red meats.

The Word speaks out on the issue of meats versus vegetable protein. It says: "And God said, Behold, I have given you every herb bearing seed, which is upon the face of all the earth, and every tree, in the which is the fruit of the tree yielding seed; to you it shall be for meat" (Genesis 1:29). The Word recommends these for meat substitutes.

Think of it! God told Adam and Eve that the vegetables and seeds could be eaten as a meat substitute. At the very dawn of history God instructed the first man and woman to live on earth that fruits and vegetables were healthier for them than meat.

I see a lot of protein deficiency among elderly people. One of the reasons is because the majority of them wear dentures and can't properly chew the meat they eat. Instead of compensating by eating legumes and grains they turn to starches and junk food.

There have been some elderly people who have come into my office who were literally starving to death. It's amazing that such a thing could take place in the land of plenty.

Lack of protein also creates poor muscle tone. That is one reason the elderly people are affected with chronic constipation. The muscle tone of the abdominal muscle and the muscle tone of the bowel become flaccid and are unable to do an effective job of pushing the bowel contents through as they should.

Protein is also used, in the formation of the autoimmune system which is a God-given ability of the body to protect itself against disease. Low immunity equals chronic disease.

Have you ever wondered why poor and elderly people are in and out of the hospital so often? It's because they don't get adequate protein in their diet.

There are a lot of elderly people who live alone and don't feel like cooking the proper foods. They may cook a good meal every two or three days and the rest of the time they snack on junk.

Many of us have been wrongly led to believe that unless we eat an abundance of red meat we may not get a sufficient supply of protein. That is untrue.

Good health requires that we limit the amount of protein we eat from the animal source. We should not eat red meat more than twice a week. This includes beef, veal and lamb. Pork should be totally avoided due to health problems associated with eating it. We should learn to eat grass-fed beef instead of the aged, corn-fed beef. We should supplement our diets with poultry such as chicken and turkey. We should limit the amount of duck or geese we eat due to the fat content.

The chicken we eat should be skinned because the skin contains the fat and also because most of the toxins in the meat are absorbed into the fat.

Baked and/or broiled fish should be eaten frequently for a good supply of protein.

I really like aged, corn-fed beef. You all know how good it is — and how fattening.

We must learn to buy cheaper cuts of meat. It will save money and cut down on the marble fat content in the meat. But we must change our eating habits to get more of our protein from legumes, grains and vegetables.

When we do this we immediately begin feeling better.

I felt bad for several years — tired, burned out and with little energy. But I changed my eating habits and now I feel excellent.

It's sheer pleasure to feel good. Whereas I used to wake up all tired out in the morning, now I get up in the morning and think, "Oh boy, another day!"

Remember that there's nothing bad about feeling good. Some may think it's just too much trouble but it all depends on a person's priorities.

Fats

Fat comes from two sources: animal and non-animal.

Fat can also be found in fish, avacado, nuts, egg yolks, milk, cream butter, vegetable oils, olive oil, peanut oil and other sources.

People often ask me: "Am I supposed to eat fats?"

"Most assuredly," I reply.

It is preferable to get the fat we eat from nuts and seeds rather than from meat.

Fats are important. They are a source of energy and also carry fat-soluble vitamins throughout the body. Vitamins A, D, E and K are fat soluble which means they can be stored in the body. Theoretically they are the only vitamins that can become toxic or accumulate in the body.

We have two kinds of fatty acids — saturated and polyunsaturated. There is a great deal of controversy among researchers on the effects they have on earth.

Saturated fats come from animals; polyunsaturated from non-animal sources.

Several years ago I attended a cardiac seminar at the University of Houston Heart Center. There we learned that saturated fats are great health hazards.

Now we have learned that polyunsaturated fats also can create health problems.

That leaves us wondering which we should use for cooking.

I personally favor corn oil which is polyunsaturated. I believe that a cold-pressed cooking oil is far superior to all others because the nutrients have not been treated out of it.

The housewife may not like cold-pressed oil because of its cloudy appearance. It is not as clear and beautiful as the cooking oil she regularly sees at the supermarket.

The housewife is to blame for the kinds of cooking oils — and other products — that are sold in the stores for if she didn't buy them the stores wouldn't sell them.

We complain about the grocers and food processors for producing food that is not good for us, with empty calories. Then, we go ahead and buy them.

We have demanded white flour because it can be stored for long periods of time.

Bugs barely bother our flour anymore. Do you know why? There's nothing for them to eat. You can hardly get a self-respecting bug to go into a bag of flour. He's afraid he will starve to death for the lack of food value in it.

The American consumer is to blame, primarily the housewife. She demands that her oil be pure so she can hold it up and see through it. But it's nothing but **trash and grease**. It has been treated to a high temperature to make it attractive. That broke down the nutrients and essentially everything good for the body was taken out.

The food industry is a multibillion dollar business and the name of the game is big bucks. They supply the housewife with what they think she wants and will buy. All of us know that they would stop producing such products if we the consumers stopped buying them.

Never use solid grease in your cooking. Grease is supposed to be liquid. Manufacturers make it solid by taking it through chemical changes at a high temperature. The catch is that the heat breaks down the molecules in order for it to remain in a solid state until heated on the stove. When it is eaten it returns to a solid state and is almost impossible to digest. It clogs up the arteries and veins and has a tremendous effect on the valves of the heart.

Numerous scientific studies reveal that fats cause heart disease by elevating cholesterol in the blood stream.

The crux of the matter is that we have too much fat and protein in our diets.

We should be neither anti-meat nor pro-vegetarian. Our goal should be one of moderation in our eating habits.

Temperance — or moderation — is one of the nine fruits of the spirit.

The Apostle Paul once wrote:

"And every man that striveth for the mastery is temperate in all things . . ." (I Corinthians 9:25).

The apostle was referring to the runners who participated in the foot races and marathons. He said in order for them to win or obtain a crown they had to discipline their bodies by not overeating. He knew that fat, unhealthy people don't win too many races.

So he recommended moderation for Christians who run in the game of life.

Red meat, chicken and fish are all good foods. But they should be eaten in moderation.

Sugar cane and sugar beets are good foods. But the food producers take those good foods through 14 processes to give the housewife beautiful, white refined sugar. She buys it because it is easy to work with. As long as she continues to buy it the manufacturers will continue to provide it.

Do you realize where the majority of the American children between the ages of three and 12 will be next Saturday morning? Watching television. Do you know what they will be watching? Cartoons. Do you know what the number one food is that is advertised on cartoons? Cereal. Do you know what one of its major ingredients is? Sugar. Do you know why your kids teeth fall out?

During my 20 years as a physician I have treated a large number of hyperactive children. It was very interesting to observe them as they bumped and jumped and twisted around in my office unable to sit still. Watching them run through my office was like watching a circus.

For years I prescribed ritalin, an amphetamine, to help calm the children. No one knows why it works so well. There were times when it calmed the children too much so we would give the children a little phenobarbitol and the children would become relatively normal. But some children got hooked on these drugs.

Now I take the hyperactive child off sugar. No cakes, no donuts, no sugared cereals. It works miracles. Ordinarily the child settles down within 72 hours. Sugar is like poison to the hyperactive child. I also restrict dyes, food coloring and additives found in processed foods from the diet of the hyperactive child.

Sugar is also poison for a person with hypoglycemia. If it is not controlled about 80 percent of the people with hypoglycemia will become diabetics.

We Americans love sugar — in candy, donuts, cakes, pies, cinnamon rolls, bear claws, danish pastries and a host of other sweet treats that delight our tastes.

Next to the French and Belgians, we eat more sugar than the people of any country in the world.

Once when I was in Brussels, Belgium, I noticed that there were chocolate shops all over the city. They make fresh chocolate every day.

While there I would get up early to take a long walk. The smell of chocolate was everywhere. Often I would see Belgian women line up at the chocolate shops waiting for them to open. Sugar is addictive and the Belgians like Americans are addicted.

Recently three women from Louisiana came to my office. They were all heavy sugar eaters and, bless their hearts, they looked like it. As part of their new nutrition program I took them off sugar, informing them that for about 72 hours they would experience symptoms of withdrawal. They didn't like the idea but accepted my diagnosis then went home.

Three days later one of the ladies called me from Louisiana.

"Doctor, I feel terrible," she said. "Am I supposed to feel this bad?"

"How bad is bad?" I asked.

"Bad bad!" she said.

"I told you it would be pretty rough for the first 72 hours," I reminded her.

"But I didn't know it would be this rough," she lamented.

After five days she called me again.

"I'm beginning to feel human again," she said.

Coming off sugar is rough because of its addictive nature. But once the transition is made it leads to improved health and a feeling of increased well-being.

Calories

A calorie is a unit in expressing the amount of chemical energy that may be released as food is metabolized.

When we say that a spoonful of honey contains 100 calories we mean that when the honey is metabolized into the body it will give that amount of energy for the body.

We Americans have become quite calorie conscious. Some people say calories really don't count but calories are the name of the game.

There is simple formula — if you eat more calories than you burn up then it goes into fat.

The three primary sources of calories are fats, carbohydrates and proteins.

Most of us gain weight for one of three reasons:

1. We eat too much.
2. We eat the wrong food.
3. Both of the above.

So for weight control and good health we must keep our calorie intake under control.

A dear lady once came into my office and said, "Doctor, I don't know why I gain so much weight because I eat just like a bird."

"Yeah," I thought to myself, "like a vulture."

A person should always be totally open and honest with the doctor for doctors know that the vast majority of overweight people just eat too much.

Cholesterol

Cholesterol is one of those red-flag words that makes us a little uneasy when we hear it mentioned. But studies show that only one-third of the American people know what it is.

It is a lipid which is a fat-like substance.

The normal cholesterol level varies according to the scale which your physician uses. Normally it is 150 to 250. But when the level increases beyond 300 these fat-like substances occlude or stop up the blood vessels. This causes stress and strain on them. Cholesterol plaque forms scar tissue and the arteries start stopping up. However, all cholesterol is not bad. There is a high-density lipo-protein which is a form of cholesterol which is good cholesterol and there is a low-density lipo-protein which is bad cholesterol. The ideal situation is to have a high ratio of high-density lipo-protein and low ratio of low-density lipo protein. Thus, through this ratio, the cardiovascular profile is greatly improved.

A certain amount of cholesterol is needed for the brain and nervous sheath.

Each person has a myelin sheath around the nerves. It is like the insulation around electrical wiring. Without it the electric current would not function properly. The nerves function the same way. Every nerve in the body has a lining of myelin which is made up partially of cholesterol.

Therefore, proper diet and nutrition are essential for proper cholesterol levels.

Glucose

Glucose is the sugar that is found in the blood. When a doctor runs a blood sugar test on you he is checking the glucose. Normally, depending on the test that is used, the glucose runs about 70-120 MG percent in the blood.

Glycogen is a type of sugar produced by the body. Glucose along with sucrose, dextrose and fructose are all broken down into glycogen by chemical processes. Then, glycogen is the type of sugar the body ultimately uses in metabolism. It then nourishes the entire body.

Enzymes

An enzyme is a complex protein that is capable of producing a chemical change.

It is a catalyst which changes other substances without itself being changed and the most important agent in the body related to chemical change.

Lipase is an enzyme that works in the inside wall of the small intestine. It performs a chemical reaction on carbohydrates but not on proteins.

All food taken into the body must be broken down

before it is absorbed.

There are thousands of enzymatic reactions on the food we eat.

Bile works on fat and breaks it down in preparation for absorption.

There are hundreds of thousands of chemical reactions taking place in your body now that you aren't aware of. No science laboratory can duplicate the complex chemical reactions in the body.

None of us say, "Well, I'm going to eat two eggs, some toast and orange juice for breakfast and my metabolism is going to function properly and digestion will follow and the enzymes in my body will change all the food I eat and I'm going to sit still and let it happen and I'll feel real good."

No, you didn't think all that. You just ate the food and in faith believed this marvelous, God-given body, would function properly.

God's Word teaches us in James 1:26:

"If any man among you seem to be religious, and bridleth not his tongue, but deceiveth his own heart, this man's religion is vain."

When most people read this verse they think in terms of bridling the tongue against gossip and backbiting.

However, it means more than that.

You can educate the taste buds of your tongue to reject bad foods. You can bridle your tongue and bring it into subjection concerning your eating habits.

Remember that the tongue controls what you swallow. Just try swallowing without using the tongue. Or try to spit without using it.

When the writer James, under the leadership of the Holy Spirit, wrote these words he was talking about a physical as well as a spiritual meaning.

If you educate your tongue to reject unhealthy foods you can control your whole body.

Try educating your tongue and see what a difference it makes in your life.

CHAPTER 6

What About Vitamins and Minerals?

A proper vitamin and mineral balance can help you feel really super good. But most people get only enough to barely exist.

It is essential that we receive plenty of vitamins, minerals and trace elements in order to have a healthful diet.

We must take vitamin and mineral supplements for three reasons.

First, most food is grown in soil that through the years has become very poor and weak. Farmers have used so much fertilizer it has stripped the soil of its nutrients.

Second, most fruits and vegetables sold in the supermarket are picked prior to maturity. They are grown in poor soil then picked green. Most of the vitamins and minerals in fruits and vegetables develop during the ripening process — on the trees or in the ground. When picked before maturity — to be shipped to the supermarket — they degenerate in quality.

Then the housewife buys these foods, places them in a pan of water and boils them. Finally, she pours them into a bowl and serves them to her family. But she is serving them dead food. Most of the vitamins and minerals — already greatly reduced when grown in weak soil or picked green — have boiled out of them.

The family would be healthier if she threw away the vegetables and fed the family the juice which remains in the pan.

That is why we need vitamin and mineral supplements.

Third, processing also depletes the vitamins and minerals in foods. You can be sure that anything on the supermarket shelf that is canned has been boiled to the point that very little food value remains. Also, food processors have added dyes, food additives, preservatives and lots of salt.

Never eat anything out of a can. If you can't buy it fresh, don't buy it.

What are vitamins?

Natural vitamins are organic food substances found only in living things. There are both natural and synthetic vitamins and I ordinarily use the natural ones.

Vitamins are formed in nature in plants, but generally cannot be produced by the human body. The body can produce vitamin K through a bacterial action in the small intestine.

Since most organic food substances, which we call vitamins, cannot be produced by the body they must be taken into the body from outside sources.

Vitamins are very valuable co-enzymes.

Remember that enzymes break down food and assist in digestion and metabolism, converting the food into energy.

When we say that vitamins act as co-enzymes we mean that they hook onto the protein molecules.

Food is broken down in the stomach and small intestine through enzymatic activity.

All cells in the body have different appearances. But they all have one basic characteristic — they must be fed to live. If they are not fed, they die.

Where do the cells get their food? From the blood supply that carries nutrients to them through the blood.

God's Word says that the life is in the blood. That is true scripturally and medically.

So, the cells have to be fed. Without adequate vitamins you cannot have the cell metabolism because the enzymes do not function properly. They act as co-enzymes.

That is a basic reason why they are so essential.

The family of vitamins includes both fat-soluble and water-soluble vitamins. The fat-soluble ones are A, D, E and K. Since these can be stored in fat they can be toxic to the body when a person takes an overdose of any one of the four.

Water-soluble ones are not toxic and if you take an overdose, they are dissolved, broken down and passed out of the body through the urine.

Now let's take a look at the functions of various vitamins.

During this discussion of vitamins I will share my daily dosage with you. But it is not a set amount. The only way I could possibly determine your needs would be to bring you into the clinic for evaluation.

Vitamin A

This vitamin is important for the health of the skin, the connective tissue in the lungs and for the little sacs in the lungs.

Adequate vitamin A gives you a good complexion. More important is the fact that it helps fight the effects of pollution in the lungs. It also assists in the formation of bones and teeth.

I personally use 25,000 international units (IU) daily. The recommended daily allowance (RDA) is far less but I recommend the larger amounts. My patients who have followed the prescribed larger dosage have shown dramatic improvement in their health.

Some of the best sources of vitamin A are liver, eggs, carrots, spinach, and broccoli.

Vitamin A is more effective when combined with other vitamins. For instance, it is much more healthful to the body when taken with B-complex. Also, vitamin C helps protect the body against any toxic effects of A.

When the A dosage is increased also increase the intake of calcium and phosphorus. And, zinc helps the body absorb A better.

Some things decrease the effectiveness of A. Mineral oil taken by a lot of elderly people, decreases the absorption of A out of the small intestine. Also, a shortage of vitamin D decreases the effectiveness of A.

Next let's examine the B-complex vitamins. These

are water-soluable and should always be taken in the correct proportions.

Vitamin B-1

This vitamin is essential for breaking down carbohydrates or carbohydrate metabolism.

Carbohydrates are a necessary source of body energy. They stablize the appetite, stimulate growth and help tone the muscles. They are particularly important for children.

A marked deficiency in B-1 can result in nerve disorders and heart palpitations. That is why the B vitamins are often called stress vitamins.

We are bombarded by internal and external stress all day long. It was a stressful situation for some of us to get out of bed this morning. We experienced stress in the morning traffic. Some people's voices even go up and down during times of stress. Poor hearing or eyesight produces stress.

So the stress vitamins are essential and B-1 is perhaps the most important.

We receive B-1 from liver, whole grains, beans, peas, seeds and nuts.

B-1 is more effective when taken with B-2, folic acid, C, E and sulphur.

You have probably heard people say, "Well, if I eat right I won't have to take vitamins." That is foolish thinking. It is totally impossible to eat correctly if you are using processed foods.

Vitamin B-2

This vitamin is also known as riboflavin. It is important for carbohydrate, fat and protein metabolism. It assists in cell respiration. Did you know your cells breathe? They do. If you don't get an adequate supply of oxygen from the blood which is carried in the red blood cells, they will die.

I recommend from 100 to 300 milligrams of B-2 per day.

It is abundant in liver, organ meat and brewer's yeast.

B-2 is more effective when taken with B-6, niacin and C.

During the summer months, when your activity increases, you should double your dosage of B-2.

Vitamin B-3

This vitamin is also called niacin and we need a lot of it.

It is used to treat heart disease for it helps to control cholesterol plaques. It is used to treat people having changes in the walls of their arteries and, in combination with other substances, we can help clear the slug out of the blood vessels.

B-3 also increases circulation and is a good remedy for people experiencing forgetfulness.

This vitamin is necessary for the metabolism of carbohydrates, fat and protein.

It helps keep the skin healthy and in certain combinations helps control acne.

I normally take about 100 milligrams per day.

Niacin is more effective when taken with B-1, B-2 and C.

Vitamin B-6

This vitamin aids in the formation of antibiotics. It also helps maintain a balance of sodium and phosphorus.

There has been a great deal of research during recent years that indicates B-6 helps prevent heart attacks.

I use it on coronary heart patients but have not used it long enough to say it prevents the attack. It has alleviated symptoms and reversed some of the heart conditions.

B-6 is more effective when taken with B-1, B-2, C, magnesium, and potassium.

Vitamin B-12

This vitamin is used primarily to treat iron deficiency anemia. It is essential for the normal formation of blood cells and helps maintain a healthy nervous system.

The best sources for B-12 are meat and animal products.

I normally prescribe 1 cc per day.

It is more effective when taken with B-6, C, folic acid, sodium and potassium.

Note that sugar breaks down the B-complex vitamins and for adequate results the sugar should be limited.

Vitamin C

This vitamin is a real wonder.

It is useful in relieving stress, helps heal wounds, and assists in the absorption of iron.

People also associate C with helping cure common colds. It has been proven very effective in treating upper and lower respiratory diseases.

Once a group of researchers set out to prove that C does not aid in treating respiratory illnesses. To their dismay, they proved it does. They didn't actually come out and say it prevents colds or other respiratory diseases. But they did acknowledge that it relieves such symptoms and reduces the amount of time necessary for recovery.

People who smoke and drink coffee break down the effectiveness of C. One cigarette destroys about 25 milligrams of C in the body. Hence, smokers have more colds.

The dosage of C can vary. Some people take as much as 15,000 milligrams daily. I recommend about 5,000 for therapeutic purposes. If you are taking a maintenance dose, about 1,000 is adequate.

Should you feel yourself coming down with an upper or lower respiratory infection or the flu syndrome, double your C or even go to 5,000. You will not become toxic. But with 5,000 you may experience some gastrointestinal discomfort for C can burn your stomach.

Good sources of C are fresh fruits and vegetables. It is more effective when taken with calcium, magnesium and all other vitamins.

Vitamin D

This vitamin is fat-soluble and is important because it improves the absorption and utilization of calcium and phosphorus which are necessary for proper bone formation. It also helps stablize nervous conditions.

Because of the PH in most people's stomachs, calcium goes through unabsorbed. D will help remedy the problem.

Since it is fat-soluble, I only recommend 800 IU per day.

D is commonly known as the "sunshine" vitamin, and is more effective when taken with A, C and phosphorus.

The main source for this vitamin is fish liver oils.

Vitamin E

This vitamin is necessary for the protection of red blood cells and for combating anemia. It also helps control cholesterol, balance the blood and keep the blood flowing.

People who have had rheumatic fever, heart damage, or a hyperintensive heart should not take E.

There are two valuable uses of E that few people know about.

It is very good in treating mastitis, or irritation of women's breasts, which is a very common disease.

I found that if these women take 400 IU daily for three weeks, the mastitis normally goes away.

Let me issue a word of caution. If any woman finds a nodule in her breast don't just say, "Well, Dr.

Whitaker said that vitamin E will cure it." Go to your physician immediately and find out what is wrong. Remember that a mass in a woman's breast is a medical emergency until proven otherwise.

A lot of people have gone through misery because they refused to pay attention to nature's warning signals. You know when you have problems. Listen to nature's way of telling your body about them.

I have treated coronary patients who developed symptoms 72 to 96 hours prior to their heart attacks. Some of them just passed their feelings of discomfort off on indigestion or shortness of breath.

Listen to the language of your body.

Also, 400 IU of E will increase the amount of high-density lipo-protein which will help protect you from heart lesions.

E is more effective when taken with A, B-complex, C, magnesium and selenium.

Sources of E include fresh, whole grain wheat products and various cold-pressed vegetable oils.

Choline

This vitamin is important for normal nerve transmission and also helps regulate the liver and gallbladder.

I normally use about 400 milligrams per day.

Choline is more effective when taken with A, B-12, C and folic acid.

Folic Acid

This vitamin is important for red blood cells formation. It also assists the metabolism of proteins.

Sources of folic acid are liver, brewer's yeast and green leafy vegetables.

It is more effective when taken with B-complex, C and pantothenic acid.

Inositol

This vitamin is necessary for formation and metabolism of fats and cholesterol. It is vital for healthy hair.

Citrus fruits and unprocessed grains are rich in inositol.

I normally use about 500 milligrams per day.

PABA

Para Amino Benzoic Acid acts in the formation of good bacteria which helps protect the body against infection.

It also serves as a co-enzyme in breaking down and utilizing protein and in the formation of nails. Researchers also have discovered it aids the protein metabolism of the hair.

It won't grow hair on a bald head but it will keep hair shiny.

PABA is more effective when taken with B-2, B-6, C and folic acid.

Pantothenic Acid

This is a stress vitamin and also affects the adrenal cortex. The adrenal cortex is where we have what is known in physiology as the flight reflex.

For instance, when you are startled you experience either fight or flight.

Pantothenic acid helps keep wrinkles away and improves the body's resistance to stress.

It is more effective when taken with B-6, B-12, C and folic acid.

This treatment of vitamins has in no way been exhaustive. My purpose is to jolt your mind and show you how important they are for good health.

Now let me share with you some helpful suggestions on how to relate vitamins to your own good health.

1. The best way to take vitamins is to start with a good multiple vitamin which includes minerals. Then add the other vitamins necessary to overcome any deficiency you may have.

You may ask, "How will I know which vitamins I need unless I'm evaluated by a doctor?"

Just listen to your body. We have outlined the symptoms which will appear if you have a deficiency.

2. If possible, come to my clinic in Texas or to some other nutritional doctor who has a medical background. The very best doctor is one who has engaged in a general practice or internal medicine and has become interested in nutrition.

You can take a whole handful of vitamins, but if you don't take them in the correct ratio they won't work well.

That is why it is hard to go into the store and buy vitamins. If you don't take them in correct proportions, they don't do you very much good.

They just pass out in the urine.

3. The very best time to take vitamins is after you eat. The reason is that vitamins can cause gastrointestinal disorders in some people.

If you are taking short-acting vitamins like C and some of the B-complexes, take them three times a day.

4. Vitamin E and iron taken together cause problems in the gastrointestinal tract. They should be taken 12 hours apart. Take the iron in the morning after breakfast and the E at night, 30 minutes before bedtime. If you don't, you will have problems.

Vitamins are so very important to good health. You don't need them to stay alive. But you do need them to feel alive.

Now let's look at some important minerals.

Calcium

Calcium is the most important mineral for the body. It helps in the formation of teeth and bones. It maintains blood clotting, helps the muscle action and keeps the body from going into various kinds of convulsions.

It is found in milk and dairy products.

The effectiveness of calcium is diminished by the lack of hydrochloric acid in the stomach.

Iron

Iron is quite helpful in fighting anemia and fatigue. Women in their menstrual periods should take large amounts of iron.

It mixes with the body's protein to form hemoglobin in the red blood cells which carries oxygen to the entire body. It also removes carbon dioxide wastes from the body.

Magnesium, Copper and Zinc

Magnesium also assists in the formation of bones and teeth as well as the soft tissues of the body. And, it helps in the metabolism of protein.

Whole grains are good sources for magnesium.

Copper helps protect the body from anemia and bone disease.

Vegetables have a lot of copper.

Zinc is important for healthy sex glands and prostate. It is found in seeds, wheat bran, oysters and herring.

Iodine and Phosphorus

Iodine is important for the production of thyroid hormones and a deficiency of this mineral can cause goiter. Sources include salt and seafood.

Phosphorus is essential for strong nerves. It assists the kidneys, and the production of hormones and teeth and bones. Sources include seafood, eggs, dairy products and most vegetables.

You must realize something about good and bad health. Your weak, run-down, tired, burned-out body condition didn't develop overnight. You slowly, gradually became the way you are by overeating, lack of exercise, junk foods, inadequate vitamins and minerals, lack of water and failing to deal with stress.

Other abuses of the body include smoking and drinking alcoholic beverages.

But body abuse accumulates over the years. And, it takes some time to put vitamins back into your body and to remedy other health problems.

If you came to me with bilateral pneumonia and were not allergic to penicillin, I would give you a shot in each hip, start you on antibiotics and would expect you to be well in seven days. I would X-ray you again in 14 days and expect all the signs of illness to be gone.

Degenerative changes in your body, brought on by years of abuse, can be reversed. But it takes time and discipline.

More than likely most of us began abusing our bodies with wrong foods when we were about six years old. For the first few years of our lives it may not have affected us so very much but eventually it catches up with us and we get sick. Then we walk into a doctor's office and say, "I want to be cured — now!"

Or, we go to the preacher and the elders of the church and say, "Anoint me with oil and pray for me. I want to be healed — now!"

God in his mercy and healing power does heal. But somehow I feel God would have been much more pleased with us if we had followed the leading of his Spirit and kept ourselves well.

There is a difference in a miracle and a healing. A miracle is what God instantly uses to get us back on the right track. But healing often takes time.

We must plant the seeds of healing with our

mouths and eating habits.

You can continually confess with your tongue that you are going to be in good health. But if you eat junk food it won't happen. God will not violate his natural laws just because you are putting trash in your body.

God is not obligated for Divine healing and health as long as we break his natural laws.

But when we follow his natural laws and take good care of our bodies then we feel much better and live much longer.

CHAPTER 7

Let's Go Shopping

Let's go shopping at the grocery store.

Sometimes when you go to the store you feel like you are going into combat.

Actually, the store owners don't like to see me coming. They know I'm going to be checking labels, comparing prices, looking for the most healthful foods and trying to get my money's worth.

Do you realize that most people, including women, don't know how to shop at the supermarket? That's unfortunate because it's true. Most of us rush into the store, grab a basket and hastily run up and down the aisles grabbing products off the shelves and throwing them into the basket.

That's a bad habit we need to break.

The first thing you need to learn about shopping is to read the labels. They contain a lot of helpful information.

"Oh, Dr. Whitaker, I don't have time to read

labels," some people tell me.

Let me remind you that you are shopping for your family and your family's health.

We're learning to shop right so that you and your family can feel better and have total health.

The label should include the name of the product and net weight. Acquaint yourself with the product and find out if the net weight is food or if it's water. Sometimes you are only buying water.

The labels should also include a list of additives in the products. Additives are bad for your health.

Artificial colorings and flavorings should also be listed. The producers are not required to name them.

We know that some dyes are carcinogenic or cause cancer. And, artificial colorings, flavorings and dyes are like poison to hyperactive children.

The Federal Drug Administration does not require the colorings and flavorings to be listed in butter, cheese or ice cream. Producers can put anything they want in these products.

Some products are known as standardized foods. These include mayonnaise and catsup which have standardized names. Producers are not required to list all the ingredients in these products. Thus they can be dangerous.

I believe that in the very near future the FDA will require that all these "optional ingredients" will be included in the labels. Then we will know exactly what we are buying.

Federal laws also require nutritional labelling — the size of the serving, the number of servings per container, number of calories per serving, and the amount of grams of protein, carbohydrates and fat.

This is very important. There are so many borderline hypoglycemics in this country. But if they watch
their intake of carbohydrates, they can have much
better health.

Sometimes you will read the word "imitation" on
the label.

What does that mean? It's not the real thing — just
an imitation of another food.

Take orange juice. If it is real orange juice and has
not been treated then it is nutritional. But imitation
orange juice is just a bunch of chemicals with water
and sugar added.

Now let's look at comparison shopping.

If you buy canned goods, which I oppose, compare
the prices of the nationally famous brands with the
brands of the individual supermarket. Sometimes you
can save up to 10 cents per can.

Why am I opposed to canned goods? Because they
have additives to preserve them and give them a long
shelf life.

The U.S. Department of Agriculture has issued the
following statement: "The majority of convenience
foods are as cheap or cheaper than those made from
scratch."

That's a bunch of baloney!

The problem with their assumption is that it is based
on cost-per-unit weight. It does not address the important subject of nutritional value.

For instance, the Department of Agriculture says
that a pound of canned or packaged stew will cost you
no more than a pound of homemade stew. They are
right so far but let's look at the contents.

Homemade stew usually contains potatoes, carrots, peas, beans and some meat. But what about the canned or packaged stew?

Usually it has unbleached flour as a filler, imitiation potatoes and simple carbohydates (sugar) added to cover up the bad taste.

You couldn't stand to eat many of these products if they were not loaded with sugar.

So the FDA is wrong to pass out that kind of information.

Have you ever read the label on one of our "fine" American foods known as cake?

Often the label will say the cake mix is "enriched." Anytime you see that word then beware. That means they have taken everything good out of it so it now must be enriched.

That is totally against God's plan for good, healthful food.

But the label will say, "enriched, brominated flour." That means bromide has been added to it. It also says the cake mix contains "niacin, reduced iron, riboflavin, sugar and animal and vegetable shortening."

The label adds that it "may contain one or more of the following: lard, cottonseed, palm oils, water, milk." Then it names some of the chemicals that have been included.

There is not one thing in them worth eating. But the American people buy them by the tens of millions.

Oh yes, packaged and canned stew and cake mixes cost about the same per unit in weight as that made from scratch. But you are buying filler. And I guarantee you that the stew will contain animal fat and products from the meat industry that they could not sell on the meat shelves. So what do they do with it? They camouflage it and put it in stew, bologna, lunch meat or some other product.

You couldn't run fast enough to catch me to give me a package or can of it.

Now let's go to the meat market.

Remember that it's all right to eat meat but we should cut down on the amount.

The less meat we eat the better health we will have. Too much fat causes cholesterol which is quite common among heavy meat eaters, people who eat meat every day.

Most supermarkets have special lighting around their meat counters which makes it very difficult to see what you are buying.

When you buy meat pick it up, turn it over, look at it and smell it. Don't be embarrassed. You are there to get your money's worth. Sometimes the meat is rancid. You can't tell just by looking at it but you can by smelling it.

A lot of people like ground meat. Do not buy pre-ground meat. Ring the bell, then pick out a piece of meat you want and have the butcher grind it up for you. Stand there and watch him grind it and then you will know exactly what you have when you get home. Make sure he runs the meat out that is already in the grinder.

Although many people don't like liver, it is a good source of iron. Make sure it comes from young animals. The reason is that when a cow is sick it is given massive doses of medicine. The antibiotics are broken down in the liver. Even if a young animal has been injected with antibiotics you have very little damage.

Veal is a good buy and a good food. So is lamb. Both are low in fat and high in protein.

Let's discuss some meats you should avoid.

Wieners — even all-meat ones — contain large amounts of preservatives. Without them they would rot. They also have a lot of coloring added. And, they are high in fat.

Poultry is a good source of protein.

I buy my chickens whole so I know exactly what I'm buying. Then, I peel all the fat away because if there are toxins in the food it will be in the fat.

Always bake, boil or roast chicken. Never fry it. It is so much better for you without white flour and grease poisoning it.

Turkey is also a good food. But avoid turkey that has a lot of fat added to it. You're just paying for extra fat that is harmful to your body.

Fish is an excellent food but don't fry it all the time. Baked fish can be prepared in a way that makes it delicious.

Why not fry fish? Because one teaspoon of lard or oil has 125 calories. The oil or grease must be about three inches deep in the skillet to fry fish.

Then what else do you add when you fry fish? Usually cornmeal, oatmeal or cracker crumbs. You know how many calories that stuff has.

What happens is that most of us take a really healthful food like fish and turn it into something unhealthful for us by the way we prepare it. We should be smarter than that.

I eat a lot of raw fish. With special sauces, it's good. Fish doesn't have to be cooked. But sometimes in July and August fish have worms. The only difference in eating it raw and frying it is that you cook the worms, too.

It is good to eat ocean fish when it is available. It has not been exposed to as much pollution as freshwater fish.

Canned tuna is excellent when canned in spring water. But watch for preservatives.

Now let's go to the vegetable shelves.

Learn to eat a lot of dried beans. They are an excellent source of protein. Soybeans are almost total protein and contain all eight of the essential amino acids.

Did you know that if you include beans, corn and brown rice in a daily family menu, your family receives all the essential protein it needs?

Soybeans have about twice as much protein as sirloin steak at one-sixth the cost.

When you learn how to make use of vegetables your health is on the way to improvement.

How do you like your vegetables? I like them raw.

If you don't like them raw then learn to steam them lightly. Thus you don't boil all the vitamins and minerals out of them.

What about milk? Raw milk is the very best but most people can't find it.

If you must buy milk make sure it is low-fat.

Powdered milk is good. Mixed with soy powder it makes an excellent drink.

Evaporated and condensed milk contain sweeteners and other additives.

When you see the word "fortified" on a milk label an alarm should go off in your mind. It means the same as "enriched." The producers have taken out of it what nature put in it. Then they have "fortified" it with chemicals.

Fruit is an excellent food. But buy it fresh. Then wash it good for often it is sprayed with harmful chemicals to keep bugs away.

Watch out for canned fruit. It has additives and preservatives for long shelf life.

When buying butter remember that slightly salted sweet butter is your best buy. Commercial butter may have undergone extended periods of storage because people play with it on the commodity market. It is not as good as fresh butter because sometimes it is made from stale milk. It usually has food coloring and additives to keep it hard.

Avoid all frozen foods which have sauces or additives used for quick preparation and long-term preservation.

Cooking should be fun and can be so rewarding.

Family health and well-being is so important. It should give a mother such great satisfaction to know she is giving her family a better life through the good food she prepares.

Many wives are killing their husbands with love. And they are doing it right in their own kitchens.

It is quite obvious that people's eating habits have run loose so long that now they are almost out of control.

I love football and parades so I enjoy going to the Rose Bowl in California.

Can you remember when the young ladies marching in the bands once were so trim and small? Last year I saw some young ladies leading bands who could play linebacker for the Dallas Cowboys.

The American people are getting fat in epidemic proportions. Some 60 to 80 million people in this country have a weight problem.

Do you want to be a part in reversing the trend?

Remember that it is impossible to have food in your house that is fattening or has empty calories unless you buy it and carry it home. If it isn't there, it can't be eaten.

Let me give you some sound advice about how to shop.

1. Read the labels. If the food has dyes, additives, preservatives, sugar, filler, grease and the like then avoid it like the plague.

2. Never go shopping when you are hungry. All the sweets will look too good to you. Get a snack before you go.

3. Never take your little children with you when you go to buy food. While you are shopping they will also be shopping for all the wrong things. When you start placing the kids' stuff back on the shelves, they will pitch a running fit and start screaming and crying. Rather than be embarrassed most parents go ahead and buy it. It's best to leave the children at home.

4. Make out a shopping list so you will know exactly what you need. That will cut down on impulse buying of those foods that look so good to you. They are usually fattening.

Remember that when you walk into a grocery store the owner is depending on you, the consumer, for his livelihood. If he doesn't give you good service by ordering the products you request, then change stores.

The battle for good health is won or lost in the kitchen where the food is prepared. It's a daily battle and has such serious consequences.

for his life-blood. If it doesn't give you good service, try ordering the product you request next chance store.

The battle of good health is won or lost in the kitchen where the meal is prepared. It's a daily battle and has such serious consequences.

CHAPTER 8

Exercise for Health — and Life

Several years ago a 70-year-old Florida man had a severe heart attack. A battery of doctors worked feverishly to save his life and it was touch and go for weeks.

Then the elderly man began to improve and he lived.

The man, still confined to his hospital bed, determined that he would change his life-style. Although he was too weak to get out of bed, he made up his mind that he would exercise his body into good shape.

A few weeks later he was able to sit up in bed. Then stand up.

He started his exercise program the first day by walking half way around his hospital bed. The next day he walked a little further.

By the time the doctors dismissed him from the hospital he was able to walk across the room and back.

The Florida man continued his exercise program for several months. He worked up to one mile, then two.

Soon he was jogging, then running. And, two years after he was dismissed from the hospital he ran in a marathon.

This story may surprise you. But it shouldn't. Our bodies are wonderfully made.

The body has such a marvelous capacity to heal itself. Bodies respond immediately to good eating and exercise disciplines.

There was a time when I hated the thought of exercise. But now that I am "a new creature in Christ" and "old things have passed away" and "all things are become new" I love to exercise. It provides a positive way I can show my appreciation to God for my body. Now my body doesn't yet know just how much I love to exercise. But it's beginning to get the message.

Some people tell me the Bible says "bodily exercise profits little."

Yeah, when the Apostle Paul wrote that he was walking 18 to 20 miles a day. He certainly didn't need an exercise program. He already had a good one.

Exercise also helps us feel better and live longer.

There is a simple formula relating to exercise: Good health requires exercise.

Good health — excellent health — is totally impossible without exercise.

The most frequent question my patients ask me is: "Doctor Whitaker, what kind of exercise program should I undertake?"

My answer is quite simple. It depends on the individual's age, physical condition and state of health regarding degenerative diseases.

Take a 40-year-old man. He can exercise more than a man who is 65, yet less than one 25.

A man or woman who is basically in good health can exercise more than those who have heart diseases or arthritis.

Yet everyone can do some type of exercise.

Before you begin an exercise program go see your doctor and ask him to give you a routine physical examination. He will advise you how much exercise your body can handle as you begin your program.

Do not exercise too much too quickly. It can kill you.

Almost everyone, regardless of age, can begin walking. Start out slowly. You older folks should begin walking one to three blocks a day. Then increase the distance a few blocks each week, or every two weeks. If you faithfully walk every day, in a few months you will be able to walk two miles a day.

It will take you about 45 minutes but will be some of the best time you spend during the day.

You should walk very briskly the first mile then slow down some as you conclude your walk.

What will you accomplish? You will be surprised how much you will enjoy breathing deeply. Many of us have a tendency to be lazy so our bodies take the course of least resistance. And the least resistance is shallow breathing.

Shallow breathing maintains life and perhaps that's all some people want. But it's not real living — it's only existing. There is a vast difference between living and existing. We Christians want to live life at its best and to do that we must exercise.

So learn to take deep breaths.

Did you know that the Word says that the life is in the blood? That's absolutely true because our bodies receive oxygen from the blood and oxygen maintains life. Without an adequate supply of oxygen every tissue in your body would die.

Medical science has determined what happens when a person has a heart attack. A blood clot forms in the wall of the heart. The reason it hurts so bad is the area of the heart beyond the clot begins to die because it is receiving no oxygen. Cardiac tissue cannot live without oxygen.

You must exercise your heart muscle for it is the most important muscle in the body.

The heart is a four-chambered muscle. When you exercise your heart improves because blood is being pumped and you start forming co-lateral circulation. That means that new vessels are being formed on the wall of the heart.

That is why the prognosis of a young man who has a heart attack is very poor. His chances for surviving the attack are less than an older man. In medicine the rule of thumb is that the younger a man is when he has a heart attack the less his chances are for survival.

The younger man does not have co-lateral circulation built up on the wall of the heart. The older we are and the more we have worked and exercised, the more co-lateral circulation we have. Then if a blood vessel gets clogged, the co-lateral circulation helps protect us. Without the circulation, if a vein clogs, we're probably dead.

Exercise strengthens your heart and all the other muscles in the body.

Let me tell you about another exercise that everyone, regardless of age, can do.

At the end of the day after you have exercised, lie flat on the floor with your feet elevated up in a chair. It does two things. It allows the blood to return to the brain and the brain to be profused with oxygen. It only takes a few minutes. This is a tremendous exercise for older people who have difficulty remembering things.

Now I'm not saying that it will make you smarter. But it will improve your memory and your overall outlook on life.

All day long blood must be pumped upwards against the force of gravity. Every day, as you sit or stand, the heart must pump blood up from your feet. But when you lie down with your feet elevated, the heart doesn't just pump the blood. It flows back down and revitalizes the brain tissue.

How long should you lie there? About 10 to 15 minutes. It can be a very enjoyable experience for you can pause and recall the events of the day.

This is a passive routine which exercises the heart. But it also gives you time to reflect on the Lord and His goodness. Try it and see how much better you sleep.

Remember that for any exercise program to be effective, it must be regular. Never exercise like a Trojan for a few days, then stop, then go back. Determine yourself what is the best program for you. Start slowly, normally three days a week. Then work up to five days and let the body rest a couple of days.

Everywhere I go people ask me about my personal

exercise program. I like the miniature trampoline and walking.

I once had heart trouble. It has been corrected through the supernatural power of God, an exercise program based on common sense and proper eating habits. Now I take long walks and regularly exercise on the trampoline.

About two minutes is plenty of time for any newcomer to the trampoline. But when you work up to 20 minutes it is the exercise equivalent to running about five miles.

Salvation and health, salvation and mind, salvation and body all go hand in hand and cannot be separated.

That is why it is difficult to have a real good spiritual walk with the Lord unless you have a strong body. You may argue the point but you cannot walk upright with Jesus and do your best for him when you feel bad. There is a definite relationship between how close a person feels to the Lord and how that person feels physically. People who are weak, tired, depressed, worn out, burned out and run down just don't feel much like a Christian ought to feel.

A good exercise program makes us stronger in the Lord and that should be incentive enough for all of us to begin a program today.

We are the last army of the Lord and in order for us to stand tall for the Master during these latter days we must be in good physical condition.

When you begin exercising give yourself some time to start feeling better. It won't take long.

Soon you will have better cardiovascular efficiency, better adrenalin flow and your vessels will begin opening up. You also will start breathing better.

All of us can practice deep-breathing exercises even while listening to the radio or watching television. Sit down on a chair, breathe deeply in and out. Start out slowly then increase the number of deep breaths. You may get a little light-headed at first. But after a time it will go away.

The major value of deep breathing is that it lowers the blood pressure. As your cardiovascular tree improves the blood vessels open up so the heart doesn't have to pump so hard to get the blood around through the body. Hence, the blood pressure comes down.

Good exercise also lowers your cholesterol and triglycerides. It accomplishes that by increasing high-density lipo-protein and thus your chances to live to a ripe old age.

I'm not just interested in your living a long life. I want you to live a good life that you enjoy. You can't do that if you feel bad.

Those with arthritis can do a limited number of exercises. If you have access to a whirlpool it would be good for any kind of water exercise makes the limbs very light and flexible.

Swimming is the only exercise that is better than walking for it exercises all the muscles of the body. Most people do not have access to swimming pools but everyone can walk.

Exercise helps relieve stress because it relaxes the body. A person in good shape also is better equipped to deal with stress when it comes. He even has a better chance of surviving an automobile accident.

It only takes two weeks of proper eating and exercise for you to look and feel better. It's worth the effort.

There are a host of other fitness plans. They include the Royal Canadian Air Force plan, calisthenics programs, aerobics, weight lifting, jogging and others. Some prefer aerobic dancing — or exercising to music — while others enjoy exercising with Richard Simmons on his TV show. Others ride bicycles.

The greatest mistake most people make in beginning an exercise program is that they want to become a Charles Atlas overnight. It doesn't work like that. It took you years to get where you are so give yourself several months of regular exercise to get where you want to be.

Plan your own exercise on what is best for you. Then do it regularly.

The goal of any exercise program is to look and feel better.

Remember that if we exercise properly, feel better and live longer there will be one less tear for God to shed.

CHAPTER 9

Sleep Is So Wonderful

Did you know that sleep is important for your good health?

It is as important as anything you do.

I know that is true for I once thought I could get by on three or four hours a night — and did for years. But it nearly killed me.

Why is sleep so important? We must have it in order for the body to repair itself after a day's work.

Each person, depending on the individual, needs a certain amount of sleep. The younger you are the more sleep you need; the older you are the less sleep you need.

The reason a child sleeps so much is because the body is developing and it needs all the energy it can get to become strong and healthy.

As we get older we normally do not work or eat as much so our metabolism is down. Thus we can get by on less sleep.

I do best on about six hours of sleep per night. More sleep than that makes me groggy and I don't function as well.

But each of you is different and should determine for yourself how much sleep you need.

Thomas Edison, the great inventor, once said a person is wasting his time if he sleeps more than three or four hours each night. But he had a secret. He took brief naps during the day. That helped renew his body.

When is the best time to sleep? At night.

God made us daytime creatures. Our best sleep is between the hours of 10 p.m. and 1 a.m. Those three hours, according to sleep researchers, are equal to six hours of sleep any other time of day or night.

According to the Word, the Creator divided time segments into day and night — the day into hours and the night into watches.

Our Lord set up a timetable whereby no meals were to be served during a 12-hour period. The first meal of the day was called breakfast or break-fast. That is why we shouldn't put anything in our stomach from about 6 to 7 p.m. to about 6 to 7 a.m.

The reason is very simple. If we eat late we don't sleep well. If we don't sleep well our bodies don't rebuild and repair themselves. God knew what he was doing.

Although people in today's shifting society sleep at all hours during the day and night, your body always knows what time it is.

Nighttime is when your sleep will be the most effective and will provide the benefits necessary for good health.

Another hint for good sleep is that you should always sleep on your back and/or right side. That is nature's way. Never sleep on your left side unless you can't sleep.

Here's why. The liver is on the right side and when you lie on your right side there is no pressure on the liver. But when you sleep on your left side, gravity pulls the liver to the left and causes it to put pressure on the aorta, the great artery coming out of the left ventricle. More people die in their sleep than any other time.

God gives us a word on when we should sleep.

We are "children of the day: we are not of the night nor of darkness" (I Thessalonians 5;5).

It is a blessing to us if we apply that verse to our lives both spiritually and physically.

Did you know that you have a biological clock in your body? And you can control that clock. Have you ever gone to bed at night knowing you had to get up at 6 a.m.? Ordinarily you woke up before the alarm clock sounded.

Sleep researchers have discovered that if we average eight hours of sleep each night we have 90-minute sleep cycles. Every 90 minutes during the night we experience rapid eye movement (REM). When you are having REM you are dreaming. It lasts from three to five minutes.

There are a number of causes of insomnia or being unable to sleep. Some of them are discomfort due to noise, inability to unwind, depression, guilt, jet lag, and poor physical fitness.

Some of the causes of insomnia are physical, some spiritual.

There are a lot of things you can do to overcome insomnia.

Take a really hot bath. That will relax you and help you sleep.

Read the Bible or some other good book for about 30 minutes prior to going to bed. That will take your mind off the cares of the day and settle you down.

A good exercise program should help you sleep better. Physical tiredness is a good antidote for insomnia. Mental fatigue is just the opposite.

The Word says: "Let not the sun go down upon your wrath" (Ephesians 4:26).

Before I was saved I often was so mad at someone that when I went to bed I couldn't sleep. I would lie there in bed and think of everything possible I could do to hurt the person. As a matter of fact, I got out of bed once or twice to go do it.

When you are mad at someone it is the last thing you think of at night and the first thing you think of when you awaken.

We must learn to forgive. We can do that through reading God's Word, meditating on it and through prayer. When we fully understand that God has forgiven us it is much easier for us to forgive others.

Do those simple things and you will sleep much better.

The sleep researchers say that we get the most benefit from our sleep from 10 p.m. to 6 a.m. The next best time is from 11 p.m. to 7 a.m.

I have yet to meet anyone who sleeps less than four hours each night who does not eventually have mood changes and become irritable.

We doctors have been trained to monitor very

carefully the sleeping habits of the elderly — say 70 or
80 years old. If we see them sleeping more than 10½
hours or less than four hours each night, we know
something is wrong, that they have a serious health
problem.

We also know that some people use sleep as an
escape and it is not confined only to the elderly. We
doctors once thought that was bad. Now we are finding that unless they do it to an extreme (pathological
sleep) then it is good for them.

But some people just go to bed and won't get up.

One of my patients was a 22-year-old woman who
did that. We got her out of bed and stood her up but
she just fell to the floor. There was nothing wrong
with her. She had just given up on life. All she wanted
to do was sleep.

Good sleeping habits seem to be a lot more important to Europeans than to Americans.

While travelling in Europe I observed that many of
them get up quite early. Usually by daybreak. They
ride bicycles — for gas is $2.80 a gallon. They eat a
good breakfast then work during the mornings. They
have a larger meal for lunch. Then they take their
siesta and sleep about an hour. They are active until
sundown and about 8 or 9 p.m. they go to bed.

But what about us? If we Americans eat breakfast
at all it consists of coffee and donuts or some other
pastry. On some university campuses you can even
see the students going to early classes drinking Cokes
or Pepsis for breakfast.

Modern man is so dumb. We drive ourselves
relentlessly all day long, eat the wrong foods and get
little exercise. No wonder we can't sleep at night.

Americans are addicted to pills. Some people must take speed when they wake up to get them going. When they get a tremor in their hands during the day they take a valium. In the evening they take another valium. By then they are so high they have to take a sleeping pill to sleep. The next morning they start the same process all over again.

Let me caution you never to take sleeping pills. If you must have them to go to sleep then something is wrong and you need to find out what it is.

There are stories in English history of how people would torture others by not allowing them to sleep. This practice exists today in China and is a severe form of torture. If a person is kept awake too long it will drive him insane.

No one can go more than a week without sleep or serious consequences will result.

Let me give you some good rules for healthful sleep.

1. Sleep with your head toward the north. This may sound a little strange to you but it is important.

We are cosmic beings. Our bodies have chemical charges. The trained eye can see these charges on the EKG printout.

The North Pole is the center of gravity. That's why the needle of a compass points north.

When I worked in the hospital emergency room I noticed that more people come in with gastric ulcers and heart attacks during the spring and fall than any other time. I can produce 17 years of records to prove that.

Also, we know that the full moon affects people, but of course not in any werewolf kind of way. .

Strange things happen during the full moon and if you don't believe it you ought to work the emergency room.

We believe we know the reason why. The body is made up of 80 percent water. What does the moon do to water? It changes the tide. It has the same effect on the body.

God formed the body out of the dust of the ground and then breathed into it the breath of life. Do you know what is left of the body after it dies? It returns to dust, to elements, minerals and trace elements we find in the earth.

We are cosmic people.

Sleep with your head toward the north and cut down on the pull from the center of gravity. Just try it and see how it works.

2. Sleep in a room which has cross-ventilation. Never sleep in a stuffy room. Turn the heat off and don't use electric blankets. Rather, use plenty of bed covers for you sleep much better in a cool, well-ventilated room. Thus, you have better health.

Recently one of my boys came home from college and said he had forgotten how cold it was in our house. He didn't spend much time in the shower.

Too much heat in a room where you are sleeping can cause all kinds of nasal, throat and respiratory problems. And, your lungs — hence your entire body — do not get the kind of oxygen necessary for good rest and healthful sleep.

3. When the weather will allow it, sleep nude. That is the way you came into this world.

Sleep nude when you can stand it — it helps you rest better.

If you can't do it, for whatever reasons, wear very loose pajamas or nightgowns to bed.

4. Sleep without a pillow.

This allows a balanced gravitational pull on the body. If the head is elevated, the pull of gravity is stronger and one does not sleep as well.

There are some individuals who have hiatal hernias and must sleep with their heads elevated. The reason for that is that if the person has an attack at 2 a.m. in the morning and is lying flat the contents of the stomach rush up into the throat.

You also should sleep on a pillow if you have fluid in the lungs, cardiovascular problems or emphysema.

5. Sleep on a firm mattress.

If you have a soft mattress, put a board under it to make it firmer.

People who sleep on firm mattresses don't suffer nearly as many back problems as those who sleep on soft ones.

6. Sleep in a dark room.

Light distracts from sleep and may startle you if you wake up during the night. You awaken, see the light and think it's time to get up. It interrupts your rest and keeps you from the ideal night's sleep.

7. Take a *siesta.*

People in Mexico, South America, France and other countries do it.

Very few Americans have ever tried it — but it works wonders in cutting down killer stress and fatigue. It just gives a person a better outlook on life.

Now don't sleep all afternoon or you won't be able to sleep at night. Just 20 or 30 minutes will do wonders for you.

8. Make a nightly review of what you have done during the day.

This helps clear the mind and prepares you for restful sleep.

Just turn off the TV, sit down in a comfortable chair and start remembering the day's events — start meditating and relive everything that took place during the day right up to the time you sat down in the easy chair to meditate.

Did anyone hurt you during the day? If so, forgive them.

A friend of mine told me about an incident with his wife. One evening she was having difficulty going to sleep because of some bad feelings she harbored against another lady in the church.

My friend suggested to his wife that she ask God to give her an inner healing of memories and take away the bad feelings. The next morning when the wife awakened she couldn't even remember who it was she had the bad feelings toward.

Or, have you hurt someone? If so, then ask forgiveness. And, if necessary, get on the telephone and make restitution by asking the person also to forgive you.

During the time of reflection, ask if you were honest with yourself during the day.

If we are to have total health we must be honest with ourselves. Pray and confess to God the wrongs you have committed against yourself, ask forgiveness and pray for deliverance.

Before you go to sleep you can rectify any negative traces in your mind just by recognizing, confessing and asking forgiveness for them.

Oh, how much better you will sleep and how much better you will feel the next morning.

9. A good walk during the day leads to good sleep at night.

If you are over 40 you may have noticed that your legs may jerk after you go to sleep at night. That is what we call the restless leg syndrome. If you walk a mile a day, the leg jerking will go away. A mile is not too far unless it's uphill.

These are some helpful hints for healthful sleep. Try them and they will work miracles in your new quest for total health.

CHAPTER 10

It Really Works!

The Prophet Daniel was one of the most fascinating men of God in the entire Old Testament. He understood Divine principles for good health.

Today he would be called a "health nut." He refused to eat the rich, sweet foods and drink the wine which he was ordered to eat by King Nebuchadnezzar.

Daniel was one of the young men carried into captivity by the Babylonians.

The Living Bible says: "Then he (the king) ordered Ashpenaz, who was in charge of the palace personnel, to select some of the Jewish youths brought back as captives — young men of the royal family and nobility of Judah — and to teach them the Chaldean language and literature.

" 'Pick strong, healthy, good-looking lads,' he said: 'Those who have read widely in many fields, are well informed, alert and sensible, and have enough poise to look good around the palace' " (Daniel 1:3, 4).

The king's men ordered the best food for them and wine from his own kitchen to help them grow strong during their three-year training period.

Daniel rejected the heavy food and wine. He knew the meats, starches, and wine wouldn't be good for his health. He realized that lots of sugar was used for making wine, and besides that he didn't drink.

So he went to the palace personnel director and cut a deal. He said he wanted to eat "pulse."

What was pulse? Historians say it included vegetables; grains such as wheat, barley and rye; peas, beans and lentils; and various seeds.

Daniel was no nutritionist but common sense and holy wisdom revealed to him that the vegetables and grains were far superior to the meat and sweets.

When he asked the personnel director if he could plan his own diet, the man replied: "I'm afraid you will become pale and thin compared with the other youths your age. And then the king will behead me for neglecting my responsibilities" (Daniel 1:10).

Daniel must have been quite persuasive for eventually the personnel director agreed to allow him to try his own diet for 10 days.

You remember what happened? At the end of the 10 days Daniel was healthier and looked better than the young men who had eaten the king's rich food.

What about Daniel's diet? It contained the essential vitamins and minerals in the vegetables; roughage in the grains; and protein in the beans and lentils.

His diet did not contain high cholesterol-producing

meats, triglyceride-producing sweets or fermented wine which would weaken his physical and mental abilities.

This kind of diet really works. It was good for Daniel and it is good for us today.

Sometime ago a beautiful 26-year-old woman came to me for help. She was from a wealthy family but had her own career as a successful fashion model.

She seemed to have everything going for her but when she came into my office she was so depressed she hardly made it through the first interview. She cried most of the time because she didn't feel good and hated herself.

The young woman had several problems. She was 30 pounds overweight and was experiencing short-ness of breath. She couldn't even walk up a flight of stairs or perform well in her work.

I told her she would have to change her life-style if she wanted to feel better. We ran the various tests to determine her state of health. Then I placed her on a sound eating program, prescribed the exact vitamins and minerals she needed to get her system back in order and suggested an exercise program. In essence, I simply showed her how to take care of her body.

She returned each month for additional sugges-tions and help.

Three months later she was a totally different woman. Today she is healthy, happy and has a new outlook on life and on her profession.

There must be tens of thousands of people like that fashion model. People who are crying, hurting and hating themselves because they feel bad.

A Christian may be the most spiritual person alive,

but if he feels bad and hates himself he won't be able to effectively serve the Lord.

One day a wealthy grain executive from Kansas came to my office. He really didn't think there was anything much wrong with him but his family insisted he visit me.

He was a little short of breath. Yet he turned out to be one of the many the Lord has sent to me who was on the verge of becoming acutely ill.

My clinic staff thoroughly examined him. We found that his blood pressure was high. His EKG revealed the left side of his heart was enlarging due to increased pressure and therefore was having to work much harder than normal to pump the blood. That caused angina or chest pains.

His cholesterol and triglycerides were dangerously high. The examination convinced me he was a borderline coronary patient.

We placed him on a strict eating plan and prescribed the necessary vitamins and minerals for his condition.

Seven weeks later he returned for a check-up. We examined him and found a remarkable recovery. The chest pains, even during exertion, were totally gone — in just seven weeks.

The man still has some heart problems. But we reduced the chances of a heart attack by changing his life-style. Actually, if he faithfully follows the program he will never have a heart attack.

That's what can be accomplished through preventive medicine. And isn't that far superior to a heart attack or open-heart surgery?

A lady with cancer and several other diseases including lupus came to the clinic. She was so sick she was unable to work. She couldn't even walk and we had to help her to the door.

After seven months of nutrition therapy, and a lot of prayer, she now is on the road to full recovery. She works from 6 a.m. to 6:15 p.m. — as my secretary.

On another occasion an arthritic cripple came to the clinic. He had rheumatoid arthritis. He couldn't move, except to shuffle his feet. And, his head was bent down. He said the ankles, knees and other joints in his body were red hot.

We examined him and found he was eating too much salt and sugar and his diet consisted primarily of junk food. He lived by himself and wasn't able to prepare good, nutritious food. And he was hurting so bad he didn't want to eat.

The different types of junk food, salt and sugar he was eating were causing a great deal of his arthritic irritation. So I recommended several changes in his eating and placed him on a vitamin-mineral program. He experienced dramatic relief from the arthritis. Over a six-month period he improved so much that he now can walk. He still has pain but is continuing to improve.

One day a renowned artist came to my office. I learned that his paintings were on display in the Smithsonian Institute in Washington and he was scheduled to have a private showing of his works in New York City.

His problem was that he had fractured the fourth and fifth lumbar vertebrae. For three months after the fracture he was unable to paint or do anything else.

Orthopedic surgeons placed him in a back brace but he still couldn't work.

We examined him and found his body was deficient in essential vitamins and minerals and his eating habits greatly contributed to the slowness of the healing process in his back.

We placed him on a good nutrition program and within 60 days he went back to painting.

Our program included regular, high therapeutic doses of calcium, vitamins A and D to aid in the absorption of the calcium and multivitamins with natural pantothenic acid. This stimulated the adrenal glands to help form calcium deposits between the vertebrae.

The therapy helped alleviate the pressure on the nerves around the vertebrae and gave him some real physical stability. He is not totally cured but is able to work free of pain.

An elderly man came to the clinic for an evaluation and examination. A previous diagnosis revealed an operation would be necessary to open the artery.

The man could hardly walk into my office. He was weak, pale, listless and felt terrible.

I put him on a good nutrition program and after a few months he is a different man. Now he is walking and doing all kinds of things. And his outlook on life is greatly improved.

The results have been incredible.

However, there are still a lot of skeptics who don't want to hear that they can feel better and live longer if they will take care of their bodies.

Sometime ago I was invited to the University of Florida to conduct a three-day seminar on nutrition and preventive medicine. Before I ever arrived there the Lord had revealed to me that it was going to be a difficult meeting.

About 15 minutes into the first lecture three women got up and walked out. A while later another four women left.

I watched them as they were leaving. Those seven women took over 1,500 pounds with them when they walked out. They just couldn't stand to hear a doctor tell them that if they wanted to be healthy and feel good they had to lose weight.

Mothers bring hyperactive children to the clinic. Hyperactivity is almost always related to sugar, junk food, dyes and additives.

Mama feeds them too many chips, dips, hamburgers and cokes. She often feeds them the quick food so she will have more time to watch the soap operas on TV.

Some mothers have brought four-, five-, and six-year-old children into my office who were so hyper they kicked their mothers in the shins and spit on them — right in my office. Yet many mothers and fathers refuse to become authority figures to their children and seldom discipline them.

A 33-year-old mother brought her seven-year-old daughter to the clinic for an analysis. The little girl was just uncontrollably hyper. The analysis revealed the child's diet was filled with junk food, additives, preservatives, dyes and sugar. No wonder she was hyper.

Do you recognize the problem? That little girl was smarter than her Mama. She could get her Mama to do anything she wanted her to do. And she ate exactly what she wanted.

That's not the way it's supposed to be — a seven-year-old telling her 33-year-old mother how she is going to act.

The mother let the child get away with it because she didn't want to hurt the little girl's feelings.

I've met other parents who are fearful that if they don't pamper their children they will not love them when they grow up.

That is pure trash. More than likely the children will grow up hating their parents because they can't respect them.

Multiply that seven-year-old girl by tens of millions and what do you have? Runaway juvenile delinquency.

I'm convinced that many juvenile delinquents are the products of two things: First, a lack of authority in the home; and second, bad nutrition which upsets the body functions and greatly influences behavior.

Remember that it's the parents who teach children how and what to eat. It's also parents who let children run wild — even in doctor's offices.

Adults come into my office so depressed they can't handle it a day longer.

Do you know what has happened to them? They don't just suddenly become depressed. They allowed it to build up for years. Then, when they allowed their bodies to get weak and out of shape suddenly they could no longer handle the depression.

Depression is an accumulation of unhealthy emotions. And it is a medical fact that a person who keeps his body in good health is much better equipped to handle the depression.

There are a number of proven ways to deal with stress, anxiety and depression.

First, get your body in shape. Lose that weight which is such a burden on your heart as well as your whole body.

Second, make sure you are eating right and getting all the essential vitamins and minerals.

Third, turn your life over to the Lord. If you really have faith in God there is never any reason to be depressed.

Fourth, you seek God by diligently learning His Word. If you do that you will have good health for His Word tells you to have good health.

You handle stress in your brain. But your brain does not function well unless your body is in good shape. If your body is strong the heart pumps adequate blood and nutrients to your brain, thus helping you fight depression.

The Word says "a merry heart" helps the body like a medicine. But a "broken spirit" dries the bones. Blood cells form in the bones. Dry up the bone marrow and it affects the blood.

I'm convinced that most disease starts in the head. The mind controls both body and life-style. It decides whether you will eat a good breakfast or bad, exercise or remain sedentary.

A lot of Christians suffering from depression come to me for help. Feelings of guilt ordinarily cause the depression.

These people know they are saved but don't realize who they are in Christ. About all they hear from the pulpits is that they are rotten, dirty sinners. So, over a period of time, they are convinced they are rotten, dirty sinners. They then develop guilt which leads to depression.

Your whole destiny depends on how you think about yourself. You must learn that as a child of God you are a supernatural individual, the actual righteousness of God, joint-heirs with Christ of everything God owns. When you come to that understanding your entire body will function better.

Another common symptom of stress is an upset stomach.

Often people come to the clinic complaining about stomach disorders.

The remedy is often quite simple.

I explain to them that after each meal there are millions of reactions taking place in the body. We really have no control over those processes but can, through anger or worry, cause those processes to become unbalanced. Then, the stomach produces a large amount of hydrochloric acid. The stomach goes into a spasm and knots up.

Often people who are experiencing tension, worry or stress will eat to try to get some relief from those strong emotions. Eating only complicates things. You should never eat when you are upset. Just drink a little milk.

The Word says we can choose between life and death. If we follow God's principles for total health we live to a ripe old age. By abusing our bodies we choose to die long before our time.

Recently a man came to my office who said he always felt bad but no one could find out what was wrong with him. He is one of those people society calls a hypochondriac. He was depressed and had a horrible outlook on life.

I suspected that he was suffering from hypoglycemia or low blood sugar. We ran a glucose tolerance test on him and monitored him every hour. The test clearly revealed he was hypoglycemic.

I placed him on the proper vitamins and minerals, suggested a new eating life-style and told him to come back for another examination in three months.

Three months later he walked into my office with a big smile on his face. His eyes were just shining and he had a spring in his step.

It was so very gratifying to see him on the road to complete recovery and feeling so much better.

In her book *How to Feel Younger, Longer* Jane Kinderleher tells the story of Lewis Cornaro, and Italian nobleman, who lived four centuries ago. She said, "His experience can guide you to a longer, happier life. . . ."

"Cornaro, you see lived 'high on the hog' — so high that doctors gave him up for an incurable invalid by the time he was 40. He had everything possible wrong with him and then some. His digestion was lousy. Any bug that was in the air, he would get. He was constantly plagued with aches and pains. His physician warned him that his only chance of surviving, even a few years longer, lay in changing his entire mode of living — immediately — at once.

"Cornaro wanted to live. He altered his eating and drinking habits and he lived in peace and health to the ripe old age of 98.

"How did he do it? He changed his regiment to one of moderation. He exercised, slept and ate at regular times — and he ate sparingly, never overloading his stomach. 'In this manner,' he wrote, 'I conformed to the proverb which says that for a man to conserve his health he must check his appetite!'

"Within a year after adopting these living habits, Cornaro was a fairly healthy man. At the age of 83 he put his formula for longevity into writing. At the age of 86 he penned a second treatise on living long. Throughout his writing he sounds a warning — do not overeat if you want to enjoy a long happy life.

'' 'I never knew any person,' Cornaro wrote, 'who ate 'til his stomach was overburdened with much food to achieve old age. Everyone would live long, if, as they advanced in years, they lessened the quantity of their food, and ate oftener, but little at a time.

'' 'Nor am I apt to be drowsy after meals,' Cornaro wrote. 'The food I take in being too small a quantity to send up any fumes to the brain. Oh, how advantageous it is to man to eat but little! Accordingly I, who know it, eat but just enough to keep body and soul together . . . oh, what a difference there is between a regular and an irregular life! One gives longevity and health, the other produces diseases and untimely death.' ''

The story of Lewis Cornaro speaks to all of us. He discovered he felt better and was healthier in direct proportion to how much, or how little, he ate.

The Word instructs us to fast or completely do without food for certain periods of time. It greatly strengthens us spiritually.

But our Lord also encourages us to fast for our health's sake — not just to punish us with hunger.

Fasting brings us excellent health benefits.

Were each of us to fast two days a week — not consecutive days — we could do away with most gastrointestinal disorders. Such a fasting program would allow the gastrointestinal system time to rest and repair itself. It would also help the cardiovascular system.

When the stomach is full the heart must pump sufficient blood to it in order for digestion and absorption to take place. When the stomach is empty, the heart gets a rest.

Remember that Jesus once fasted 40 days. Researchers have discovered that during the first 40 days of a fast the body draws on fat or eats up fat for energy.

About the fortieth day starvation begins and the body starts eating itself or its protein.

The Word is quite medically wise.

Divine health principles really work! They can help you feel so much better and live a lot longer. The success of any such program is based on how much better you feel.

But the choice is yours.

CHAPTER 11

Hope Without Surgery

Now I want to share something very exciting with you.

There has been a great breakthrough in the treatment of heart disease. It is called Cardiovascular Chelation and has proven to be very effective in the treatment of arteriosclerosis (occlusive vascular disease).

It is a proven treatment that offers hope without surgery to many heart patients.

Chelation — pronounced kee-lation — is a form of therapy aimed at reducing calcium deposits in the arteries and other parts of the body. The treatment involves injecting small amounts of an amino acid — Disodium Ethylenediamine Tetracetic Acid (EDTA) — into the venous bloodstream.

EDTA has the unique and valuable property of being powerfully attracted to ionic calcium. When EDTA comes in contact with ionic calcium in the body it binds itself to it. This is similar to pulling rivets out of a bridge. Without the rivets the bridge collapses. The EDTA calcium complex is then excreted through the kidneys and passed in the urine while the fats and cholesterol from the hardened artery are altered in the liver, and passed out through the gastrointestinal tract. Thus, this binding property of EDTA provides the basis for chelation therapy.

The word "chelate" is derived from the Greek word *chelos* which means to claw out. There is a pincer-like binding of certain chemical substances to bivalent metals or other minerals. Chelation is defined as the incorporation of a metal or metallic ion into a heterocyclic ring structure.

Certain chemicals are used in chelation to grasp metals or calcium with this claw-like action so that these metals are encircled by a complex ring structure, thus losing their physiologic and toxic properties. Hence, when chelation occurs, the calcium or heavy metal comes in contact with a chelating agent, becomes imprisoned in the chelating agent, and is excreted from the body in bond, inert form.

The Chelation Process in Nature

In nature, chelation is one of the most important functions taking place. In the bodies of living organisms, both animal and plant, it is the means by which inorganic minerals are utilized. It is a marriage of the organic chemical world with the inorganic chemical world. Chlorophyll, the green portion of plants, is a chelate of magnesium.

Hemoglobin, the oxygen carrying pigment of red blood cells, is a chelate of iron. The chelation process is involved in the formation and function of enzymes, which are the protein substances controlling most of the vital functions of the body.

Some of the successful medications used in the treatment of diseases are dependent upon chelation for their action, including vitamin C and E.

Chelation processes are some of the most complex chemical reactions found in nature and control many body functions. The same principles are used in cardiovascular chemotherapy to treat arteriosclerosis, cerebral and stroke, coronary heart disease and artery diseases of the lower extremities, arthritis, heavy metal poisoning and even poisonous snake bites. The same principles also apply to psoriasis and scleroderma.

Chelation: Uses in the Treatment of Disease

Chelation therapy originated in Detroit, Michigan, in 1949 as a result of the observations of the Doctors Norman, father and son, who were using EDTA to treat lead poisoning. Lead was removed from the bloodstream and other body storage areas by means of an intravenous infusion of EDTA. It was observed that patients who had lead poisoning and arteriosclerosis began to improve markedly following chelation with EDTA. The improvements were related to the symptoms of arteriosclerosis as well as those that resulted from lead poisoning.

In the history of chelation, one sees that experimentation and usage by various investigators resulted in the development of techniques for the successful treatment of the catastrophic effects of arteriosclerosis involving the lower extremities, brain and heart, as well as the general arterial circulation of patients. Clinical usage of chelation in the treatment of disease processes has since been developed by numerous physicians working with thousands of patients using EDTA without a single reported fatality due directly to the treatment.

Excellent results have been obtained in the treatment of arteriosclerosis, sclerotic heart valves, coronary heart disease, intermittent claudication (leg pains due to lack of circulation), impending gangrene, angina pectoris, heart attacks, strokes, senility, scleroderma, arthritis, degenerative joint disease and psoriasis. Studies have shown that the basis of most of the problems is poor circulation caused by hardening of the arteries or calcinosis.

Chelation therapy has consistently shown a definite improvement in the circulation of patients as evidenced by improvement in skin color, arterial pulsation in the feet, return of normal temperature in the feet, restoration of the ability to walk long distances comfortably, elimination of anginal (heart) pain, improved brain function and improvement of muscular coordination.

Additional benefits are often improvements in hearing and vision. Chelation also generally results in a significant improvement in coronary circulation, in most cases to the extent that the cardiovascular chemotherapy has been found to improve kidney function and reduce prostatic obstruction; and produces significant improvements in arthritis, and some improvement in patients with multiple sclerosis.

Most patients also have increased energy and

improved tactile sense.

Arteriosclerosis — Hardening of the Arteries

Arteriosclerosis is the number one killer in the United States today. In 1973 alone, an estimated one million persons died in this country due to the consequences of this disease.

In the United States some 54.6 percent of the deaths result from arteriosclerotic disease. This does not include the 13 percent who die from strokes.

Cancer causes 13 percent of the annual deaths.

However, arteriosclerosis is the leading cause of death in all patients over 35, black men over 45 and black women over 35.

There are several different types of arteriosclerosis, the most common form of which is atherosclerosis. Hardening of the arteries, regardless of the type, results in a narrowing or stenosis of blood vessels and may affect any or every part of the body. Some of the most serious disease entities include coronary heart disease, stroke, hypertension, diabetes, kidney disorders, senility, thyroid and adrenal disturbances, emphysema and Parkinsons Disease.

The basic problem is decreased arterial blood supply to the organs and failure to deliver adequate nutrients and oxygen. Disease of the organ, and ultimately death, are the end results.

Arteriosclerosis, although usually associated with aging, may begin in early childhood. It is not until the cross sectional area of the blood vessel is reduced by more than 70 percent of normal that significant changes are noted; even up to 50 percent reduction is tolerated fairly well by the body. It is because of this tolerance that younger people function without clinical symptoms of the disease. Unfortunately, the average diagnostic tests usually fail to reveal the true disease state of many patients.

The arteries are primarily affected in arteriosclerosis. An artery is composed of three basic layers: an inner layer known as the *intima;* a middle muscular layer, the *media;* and an outer layer known as the *adventitia.*

In the case of arteriosclerosis, yellowish plaques (atheromas) develop within the *intima* of the larger and medium-sized arteries. These atheromatous plaques contain cholesterol, fatty material (lipids), proteins, polysaccharides, and minerals (usually calcium).

Another form of arteriosclerosis is mockebergs, in which deposits of calcium develop within the *media* of the larger arteries. Cardiovascular chemotherapy attacks arteriosclerosis by acting primarily on the metallic elements of diseased arteries.

Calcium in the human exists in several forms. In the bones and teeth, calcium is firmly bound to protein and other molecules and is not easily removed by chelation. However, part of the calcium is in a readily available ionic form.

The level of this ionic calcium in the blood serum is rigidly controlled by the parathyroid glands. As calcium is removed from the serum by chelation, it is also pulled out of the other areas of the body in order to maintain a constant serum level.

The most accessible form of calcium is in those areas where it has been abnormally deposited — from the inner walls of the arteries, around tendons, joints, ligaments, kidneys, pancreas and skin. These abnormal calcium deposits are referred to as metastatic calcium deposits or pools, and consist largely of ionic calcium, a form similar to that found in the serum. Thus, abnormal areas of calcification can be gradually reduced over a span of time.

However, calcium is not the only material present in the atheromatous plaques of an arteriosclerotic artery.

The atheroma also contains other metals, and some of these are removed along with the calcium. The calcium and other minerals tend to act as cement binders and when these metals are removed the remaining material consisting of cholesterol, lipids, proteins and polysaccharides begin to break down slowly into solution. The calcium and other minerals which are bound to the EDTA pass through the bloodstream and are excreted within the urine by the kidneys.

Microscopic particles and molecules of the other portions of the atheroma are consumed by macrophages in the blood stream, blood flow is increased and the arterial circulation of the patient is improved.

A physical law states that an eight-percent increase in arterial diameter results in two-fold increase in blood flow if a laminar flow, or a four-percent increase results in a two-fold increase if a turbulent flow.

EDTA is akin to aspirin in that not all of the mechanisms by which it exerts its beneficial effect are presently known. In addition to the chemical binding of heavy metals and calcium ions, it appears that other systems and processes are affected. The quick response of angina pectoris patients, the improvement of stroke victims, the delayed beneficial results up to several months after treatment, especially in increased energy and improved tactile sensation which occur after treatment, the improvement in blood lipid values and many other restorative improvements strongly suggest that EDTA has a greater spectrum of useful therapeutic activity than is currently understood.

In chelation therapy the improvement in arterial circulation is not limited to the effects of EDTA but is enhanced by an intensive nutritional program which accompanies the chelation. Cardiovascular chelation is also augmented by the proper use of adjunctive modalities which yield the excellent therapeutic results.

Chelation with EDTA should be considered in any disease in which there is decreased blood supply and/or abnormal deposits of free ionic calcium present.

The efficacy of the therapy varies with the disease process, the degree of severity in the individual and the cooperation of the patient.

Cardiovascular chelation should go along with a complete change in health of the patient. Anyone unwilling to make a complete commitment to developing good health habits should not consider taking this treatment.

It is difficult to accurately predict the extent of chelation treatment's success in any specific case. However, clinical data based on the experience of many physicians over a period of almost two decades, involving hundreds of thousands of treatments, indicate that a positive response with excellent results occurs in about 80 percent of the patients. An additional 15 percent show good improvement, and five percent of the cases show little clinical evidence of improvement.

Cardiovascular Chelation: Do You Qualify?

Before cardiovascular chemotherapy can be started the patient must be carefully evaluated. This includes a complete history and physical examination, complete blood count, chemistry profile, urinalysis studies, chest X-ray, electrocardiogram, Doppler vascular studies, hair and diet analysis, thyroid studies.

Certain other studies, such as electrocardiographic stress testing may be required in specific cases.

Particular attention is directed to the lungs, kidneys and liver. Patients having old calcified tubercular lesions in the lungs are usually not acceptable for cardiovascular chemotherapy. To eliminate calcium resulting from chelation the kidneys must be functioning properly. Persons suffering from kidney or marked liver dysfunctions are usually not acceptable for cardiovascular chelation.

The golden age for preventive medicine and cardiovascular chelation is the late 30s, 40s, 50s, 60s and even into the 70s.

Although cardiovascular chelation is commonly used as a therapeutic modality, it is most effective as a preventive measure. Chelation prevents some of the more serious catastrophic events associated with arteriosclerosis. An ounce of cardiovascular chelation prevention is better than a pound of chelation cure.

Look at these astounding facts:

• There have been no deaths from chelation therapy in over 25 years.

• There have been no serious side effects in our office.

• There has been an 80- to 90-percent success rate.

Every medical therapy involves some degree of risk and chelation is no exception. Although hundreds of thousands of treatments have now been given without lethal, untoward reactions, the patient should be informed of the potential risks involved.

But I believe that when EDTA is properly administered by a physician by slow intravenous drip in proper concentrations, it is essentially non-toxic and generally can be promptly controlled. Too rapid an infusion may cause an aching, which extends up the arm to the shoulder and chest. This is why the treatment is administered very slowly. Other side effects may occur, but are infrequent.

The minor side effects are minimal when compared with the catastrophic and death-dealing effects of the non-treatment of arteriosclerosis and the consequent severe heart attacks, severe strokes, loss of limbs due to gangrene. The beneficial effects seen in the past 25 years are tremendous and many times astounding.

Let me recommend that you read a book entitled *Chelation Therapy* by Dr. Morton Walker if you want further information on this extraordinary treatment. It contains numerous testimonials by chelated patients and gives information and insight to chelation's history and the barriers by "orthodox" medicine with which chelating physicians have had to cope and overcome.

About the Author

Dr. Donald Whitaker is a successful physican and surgeon. He also is:

• The founder of the Orthomolecular Clinic in Longview, Texas.

• A former teacher of microbiology at Texas Christian University in Fort Worth, Texas.

• A former nuclear physicist.

• Host of his own television program each week on the Trinity Broadcasting Network in California. The name of the program is "Calling Dr. Whitaker."

• A health seminar teacher and lecturer throughout the United States.

• A speaker for churches, Christian television talk shows and Full Gospel Businessmen's meetings.

Dr. Whitaker graduated from Kansas City College of Medicine and Surgery and did an internship and advanced work in surgery at Hillcrest Hospital in

Oklahoma City.

While in private practice, he had one of the most successful medical practices in the State of Oklahoma.

In February of 1975 Dr. Whitaker came face to face with death. His experience during that time of severe crisis revolutionized his life. When the Lord Jesus Christ came into the life of this Oklahoma doctor He brought with him healing of body, soul and spirit.

After receiving Christ, for the first time in is life he was no longer plagued with an insatiable, tormenting vacuum inside his very being. God had graciously healed him and put joy in his heart.

This miraculous conversion and healing changed not only his life, but his medical practice as well. The words found in Hosea 4:6 rang out in his spirit: "My people are destroyed for lack of knowledge. . . ." Consequently, Dr. Whitaker opened the Orthomolecular (Preventive Medicine) Clinic in Longview, Texas.

Dr. Whitaker travels throughout the nation ministering to the total person — spirit, soul and body. He also conducts health seminars throughout the country teaching the Wholistic principles of living.

God has called Dr. Whitaker to educate his people in caring for their bodies.

He often quotes the Word of God which asks: "Do you now know that your body is the temple of the Holy Spirit who is in you, whom you have from God, and that you are not your own? For you have been bought with a price; therefore, glorify God in your body and in your spirit . . ." (I Corinthians 6:19, 20).

According to Dr. Whitaker, H.E. Sigerist, one of medical society's most eminent historians, commented: "The ideal of medicine is the prevention of disease."

Dr. Whitaker says that Orthomolecular Medicine is essentially the treatment and prevention of disease by the expert adjustment of the natural chemical constituents of our bodies. Each individual is biologically unique and may have unusual needs, sensitivities or intolerances that express themselves as symptoms. The proper assessment of these needs and the provision of the right nutrients (molecules) in the proper amounts is Linus Pauling's definition of Orthomolecular Medicine.

Although this particular branch of medicine is considered to be in its infancy by the traditional medical world, Dr. Whitaker says we find the words of the Yellow Emperor, Huang Ti, declaring, "The superior physician helps before the early budding of a disease." This statement was recorded more than 4,000 years ago. Physicians are finding that good nutrition plays an essential role in the maintenance of health and particularly in the recovery from acute illness or injury.

Dr. Whitaker says the Word of God is a vast reservoir of information emphasizing the aspect of Preventive Medicine. When he first became interested in Preventive Medicine he looked around him and saw a society that indulged in excessiveness. He also saw the basic biblical principle of "Whatsoever a man soweth, that shall he also reap," being exemplified in people's lives.

He determined, with the guidance of the Holy

Spirit, to educate the people by presenting the latest knowledge available to him on maintaining good health, improving poor health and caring for the total person — spirit, soul and body — so that each might live the kind of victorious life that God intends for his people to live, free of pain, suffering, depression and despair.

According to Dr. Whitaker, it is up to each individual to make a decision to BE WELL, otherwise all of the knowledge and skills available to mankind will not bring one to a state of continual health. Once this decision is made, a person is on the road to total health, the ultimate in Preventive Medicine.

Dr. Whitaker's clinic in Longview, Texas, is an out-patient facility dedicated to the Orthomolecular principles of medicine. The clinic's staff works as a team to conduct the necessary tests with the least amount of inconvenience and discomfort to the patient.

The preliminary procedures for those visiting the clinic include the following:

1. An in-depth analysis will be made of each patient's nutritional habits. For seven days prior to the initial visit, each patient must maintain an accurate diary of everything taken by mouth (with the exception of water).

2. Each patient must fast for 10 hours immediately preceding the laboratory analysis on the initial visit. (Water is absolutely the only thing taken by mouth during the fast period.)

On the first day of the initial visit, each patient receives a chemical assessment which includes an extensive series of laboratory tests which examine the natural chemical constituents of the body.

Following the chemical assessment, a computer analysis is made. Through the technology of Computer Science, Dr. Whitaker is able to accurately analyze the foods eaten and determine basically what nutrients are in those foods. The computer analysis provides a wealth of information enabling a more efficient means of accurate patient care. This service does NOT serve as an alternative to traditional patient care, merely an additional service available in caring for the patient.

Dr. Whitaker also does an in-depth study of the patient's physical and medical history. Through that study he receives the information needed in solving complex problems as pertinent information in the patient's nutritional and medical history is detailed.

According to Dr. Whitaker, it is helpful if patients can list, in advance, any major illnesses, injuries, familial diseases or surgeries and their dates.

After a thorough evaluation, Dr. Whitaker discusses the findings of the analysis with the patient and recommends the appropriate treatment.

Anyone who wants further information should write Dr. Donald Whitaker, 1800 Judson Road, Suite #7, Longview, Texas 75601, or call (214) 758-3990 or 758-3989.

This book is available at the following prices:

QUANTITY	DISCOUNT	PRICE EACH
1-10	None	$4.95
11-24	10%	4.50
25-49	20%	3.95
50-99	30%	3.50
100 +	40%	2.95

Order from:
HUNTINGTON HOUSE, INC.
1200 N. Market Street, Suite G
Shreveport, Louisiana 71107
(318) 222-1350

ORDER BLANK

Please mail _____ copies of **Nature's Kitchen** to the following address; enclosed is my check/money order for the total: **Nature's Kitchen,** P.O. Box 1117, Lufkin, Texas 75901.

_____ copies @ $11.97 each. $11.97 × _____ = _____

_____ postage & handling fees @ $2.00 each.

$2.00 × _____ = _____

_____ 5% state sales tax (Texas residents only)

$.60 × _____ = _____

TOTAL . . . . . = _____

NAME _____

ADDRESS_____

CITY _____

STATE _____ ZIP _____

HOUSE CALLS

The Monthly Nutrition Newspaper for the Layman

$24/YEAR [12 ISSUES]

NAME _____

MAILING ADDRESS _____

CITY _____ STATE _____ ZIP _____

HOUSE CALLS / Donald R. Whitaker, D.O.
1800 Judson Road, Suite 7 • P.O. Box 4177
Longview, Texas 75601   [214] 758-3990

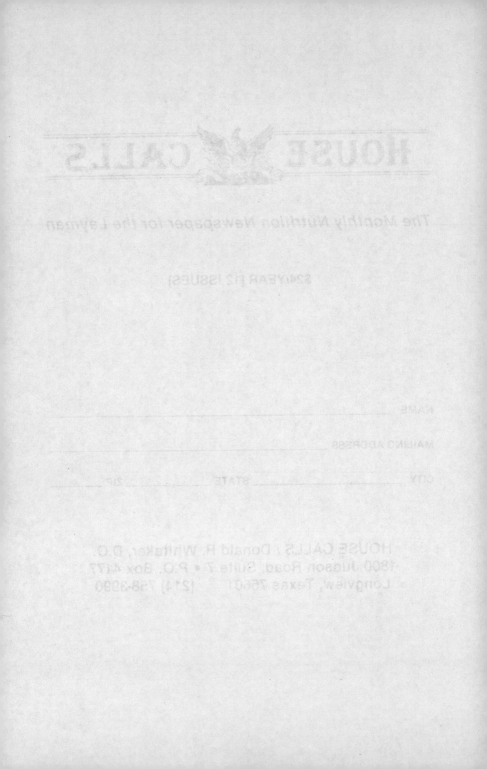

Don't Miss These Tapes

Please send the following:

- ☐ *What You Have Asked & What You Want to Know*
  Set of 4 Tapes $16.00
- ☐ *How to Have Total Health (Seven Steps to Divine Life)*
  Series of 10 Tapes $40.00
- ☐ *Cancer & Prevention* One Tape $4.00
- ☐ *Hypoglycemia — Prevention & Treatment* One Tape $4.00
- ☐ *Good News Tape (Jesus Christ Lives & That's Good News)*
  One Tape $4.00
- ☐ *Personal Testimony* One Tape $4.00
- ☐ *Heart and Cardiovascular* One Tape $4.00

Send to: **Born Free Evangelistic Association**
Dr. Donald R. Whitaker
1800 Judson Road, Suite 7
P.O. Box 4177
Longview, Texas 75601

I am enclosing $ _____

Name_____

Address_____

City_____

State _____ Zip _____

I am enclosing $ _____

Name_____

Address_____

City_____

State _____ Zip _____

Yes! Please send me information on FANAFI Food Supplements and on CORNERSTONE Natural Food Products.

MY NAME _____

MY ADDRESS _____

CITY _____ STATE, ZIP _____

PHONE _____

TO: Dr. Donald R. Whitaker
      1800 Judson Road, Suite 7
      Longview, Texas 75601

Yes! Please send me information on FANAFI Food Supplements and on CORNERSTONE Natural Food Products.

MY NAME _____

MY ADDRESS _____

CITY _____ STATE, ZIP _____

PHONE _____

TO: Dr. Donald R. Whitaker
      1800 Judson Road, Suite 7
      Longview, Texas 75601

NATURAL PRODUCTS *for You!*

Natural vitamin supplements and food products are necessary for your good health and nutrition. Dr. Whitaker long ago recognized this need and proposed to fill it. Thus, FANAFI* SUPPLEMENTS were created to bring you the most current and balanced formulations available.

And complimenting FANAFI SUPPLEMENTS are CORNERSTONE NATURAL FOOD PRODUCTS. Now being specially developed for your use are healthy and nutritious staple and convenience foods. These will include easy to prepare entrees, soups, snacks, dehydrated fruits and vegetables, whole grains, beans, nuts, seeds and other items.

Continuing research and product development in both FANAFI SUPPLEMENTS and CORNERSTONE NATURAL FOOD PRODUCTS will help insure your good health today and in the days ahead, naturally.

Find a Need and Fill It.

For further information please fill out and send the request card provided or write:

Dr. Donald R. Whitaker
1800 Judson Road, Suite 7
Longview, Texas 76501

GIFT IDEA

I want a gift copy of **Nature's Kitchen** to be sent to the following people to share the life-changing power that is ministered through this book:

NAME _____

ADDRESS_____

CITY _____

STATE _____ ZIP _____

NAME _____

ADDRESS_____

CITY _____

STATE _____ ZIP _____

NAME _____

ADDRESS_____

CITY _____

STATE _____ ZIP _____

I have enclosed a check/money order for the total:

_____ copies @ $11.97 each. $11.97 × _____ = _____

_____ postage & handling fees @ $2.00 each.

$2.00 × _____ = _____

_____ 5% state sales tax (Texas residents only)

$.60 × _____ = _____

TOTAL . . . . = _____

Gift card from _____